A Paradigm-Shift
in Pain Medicine

A Paradigm-Shift in Pain Medicine

Implementing a Systematic Approach to Altered Pain Processing in Everyday Clinical Practice Based on Quantitative Sensory Testing

Doctor of Science Thesis by

Oliver H.G. Wilder-Smith

Center for Sensory-Motor Interaction, Department of Health Science and Technology, Aalborg University, Denmark

River Publishers

Aalborg

ISBN 978-87-93102-55-2 (paperback)
ISBN 978-87-93102-54-5 (e-book)

Published, sold and distributed by:
River Publishers
Niels Jernes Vej 10
9220 Aalborg Ø
Denmark

Tel.: +45369953197
www.riverpublishers.com

To Elly with love and thanks

Psalm 19

This manuscript is the basis of my doctor of science dissertation at Aalborg University, Denmark, defended on September 27, 2013 and approved by the Academic Council on October 25, 2013.

Contents

Preface

A work like this is never possible alone. I was supported by many people in my quest to understand the link between changed central pain processing and better management of chronic pain. It would not have been possible for me to realise my quest without the input, discussion, critique and multidisciplinary expertise which the collaborations that I was privileged to enter into over the years provided. In the following – non-exhaustive – list, I would like to pay tribute to some key persons who accompanied and supported me in this project.

Geneva University Hospital in Switzerland was the place I started my pain research. Edömer Tassonyi, with whom I worked in the Anaesthesia Unit for Head Surgery gave me the enthusiastic support and advice essential for starting up my first research projects involving quantitative sensory testing (QST) after surgery. These projects would never have been realised without the tireless help of my colleagues at the department, such as Claude Senly and Dorothee Gaumann, in gathering data from the surgical patients.

For one of the pioneering conferences on pain and surgery Edömer and I organised together in the early 1990s at Geneva, I invited Lars Arendt-Nielsen from the Centre for Sensor Motor Interaction (SMI) at Aalborg University, Denmark, to speak. A pioneer of the use of QST in experimental human pain research, he rapidly became a key long-term collaborator in my quest to apply QST for clinical pain research. Since then his enthusiasm, expertise and stamina have been a driving force for our many joint research projects, crucially contributing to the innovation and success of our studies. I have always enjoyed our close interactions over the years, and I fondly remember my time at the SMI in 2007 as visiting professor.

A short time after getting to know Lars I encountered a colleague of his from Aalborg, Asbjørn Drewes, at a meeting on a new topic for me: visceral pain. His unique proficiency in – and passion for – the field of visceral pain and its study via QST and EEG proved irresistible. We also discovered another shared interest, good food, leading to many productive brain-storming restaurant sessions together at conferences where we both happened to be speakers. Later on, we started to seriously collaborate on research into a further shared passion, pain in chronic pancreatitis, and this became another reason for regular trips to Denmark. The times I spent together with Asbjørn's research team at Mech-Sense are memorable, as are the unique Danish PhD defences in which I was honored to be opponent.

My long-lasting and close collaboration with my Danish friends is – and will continue to be – a great source of inspiration for me and my research into altered pain processing and its relation to pain diseases.

Another person I invited to speak at a Geneva conference was Ben Crul, a pioneer in the development of clinical pain medicine in the Netherlands. Closely associated with the setting up of EuroPain, an early European group initiating and supporting collaborative pain research, his interest proved infectious and I was soon recruited to this cause, initially as board member, and later on to succeed Ben as president. Ben's recruiting abilities did not end there, however, and at the beginning of the 21st century he persuaded me to join him at the Clinical Pain Unit of the Department of Anaesthesiology, Radboud University Medical Centre in Nijmegen, The Netherlands, to help set up a programme of pain research. He introduced me to the world of structured, professional, academic and multidisciplinary clinical pain practice covering acute, oncological and chronic benign pain, while advising and lobbying enthusiastically regarding my pain research up to his retirement a few years later. I much appreciate the personal support Ben provided during my early years in Nijmegen, and for the energy and zeal he has continued to invest into the cause of developing clinical pain practice and research.

Shortly after starting at Nijmegen, I was introduced to an energetic general surgeon, Harry van Goor, who – I was reliably informed – was also interested in pain. On getting to know Harry, I discovered that he was not only genuinely interested in pain, but that he was seriously interested in chronic pancreatitis. This combination proved difficult to resist, and I was soon involved in helping supervise the first of what was to become a line of PhDs investigating the field of chronic pancreatitis and pain. Fueled by Harry's involvement in the Dutch Pancreatitis Group, we started up a systematic research programme to understand the impact which chronic pancreatitis has on central processing. This line was soon reinforced by Asbjørn and his team. Since then, our collaboration has gone on to publish cutting edge, internationally recognised innovation in our understanding of the mechanisms underlying chronic pain in the context of chronic pancreatitis. The close association with Harry continues to be one of the main engines driving my pain research and its development.

When Ben Crul retired, he was succeeded by Kris Vissers, a specialist from Belgium in palliative care and pain medicine. Kris was preceded by a reputation as a talented medical administrator. Despite our different backgrounds, we discovered that we shared an zest for innovative medical research and its implementation in clinical practice with the goal of quantum-shifting its effectiveness for the patient. This discovery became the basis for an effective, long-term collaboration to transfer diagnostic methods revealing altered central processing in chronic pain from the laboratory to everyday clinical practice. Implementing a suitable QST system into clinical practice was key to this project. Thanks to Kris' enthusiastic support, our Department has become the first worldwide to implement QST in regular, routine clinical pain practice in the form of the Nijmegen-Aalborg Screening QST (NASQ) presented in this thesis. With the support of Gert-Jan Scheffer, the Head of the Department of Anaesthesiology, the NASQ is now also finding its place in perioperative screening for risk of unfavourable pain outcomes after surgery. The complementary relationship Kris and I have developed will continue to be a bedrock of our ongoing research, development and clinical implementation programme to achieve pioneering QST-based systematic approaches to chronic pain management.

An onerous and ambitious research programme such as the one presented in this thesis would not be possible without the talented and hard-working PhD students I have been privileged to supervise during my time at Radboud University Medical Centre. My warm and heartfelt thanks go out to André Wolff, Monique Steegers, Jan Oosterhof, Antoinette van Laarhoven, Hessel Buscher, Emanuel van den Broeke, Nicholas Chua, Stefan Bouwense and Hans Timmerman for their enthusiastic and dedicated contributions to our pain and QST research programme.

Last – but certainly not least – I would like to thank my wife Elly for her constant, dedicated, enthusiastic and wise encouragement from the moment this project was born. You never doubted the necessity and usefulness of implementing QST to radically transform clinical pain practice. Your proof-reading was always of the highest standard. Even in times of discouragement you never ceased to have faith in my ability to crack this nut! With much pleasure I remember our many stimulating discussions, arguing the pros and cons of the research and its presentation – and (always your strong point) how to make it impact reality by improving the daily life of the patient. Without your patient and persuasive backing this thesis would not yet have seen the light of day! Thank you for being my opposite in the process of conceiving and writing this project, for your unwavering belief in my vision of better pain patient management, and your ongoing support in matters of daily living during the period of putting the thesis to paper.

Foreword

The development of generalized sensitization during acute pain conditions plays an important potential role for the transition to and development of chronic pain. Such a phenomenon complicates adequate pain management and challenges current therapeutic modalities. This doctoral thesis aims to investigate the application of quantitative sensory testing in a clinical setting, mainly postoperative pain and chronic pain states. The pathophysiology, extent, and intensity of generalized sensitization, and in particular its relation to clinically relevant patient experiences, i.e. spontaneous pain and pain evoked by daily activities, are still a matter of debate and intensive research. The current thesis has taken on the difficult task of applying standardized quantitative sensory testing to clinical medicine to explore the extent and magnitude of sensory perturbation in a number of important conditions.

The thesis is a very impressive and pioneering collection of important pieces of research providing a strong assertion on how pain can be diagnosed and profiled. It comprises an important contribution to the progress of the field and the impact of the studies will pave the way for new explorative studies for the benefit of patients suffering from chronic pain. Going from a purely descriptive way of thinking, the thesis has developed, in an ambience of changing concepts in pain medicine at large, a shift towards a mechanism-based way of thinking. This is the only way to make a step forward in pain medicine both when it comes to understanding the complex pictures presented by pain patients, and to provide clever answers to the complex therapeutic needs of these patients.

The scientific work described in this thesis is original, and the findings contribute to new and better understanding of the pain syndromes investigated. This work also provides important information for planning future research.

I have known and collaborated with Oliver since the early 1990s, and he is a true pioneer within the research to apply QST in the clinical setting. Therefore, I was extremely honoured when he chose to submit and defend his doctor of science thesis at the Center for Sensory-Motor Interaction, Aalborg University, and I am very much looking forward to our future collaboration and interaction in many years to come.

Lars Arendt-Nielsen

Executive Summary

Pain persisting beyond tissue healing after trauma and ensuing chronic pain syndromes continue to have a major personal and societal medical impact. Despite intense and concerted efforts in the last decades at achieving effective management through scientific and organisational advances, little real impression has been made by present symptom-based therapeutic approaches on the prevention and treatment of chronic pain. Thus chronic pain and its development is a common, clinically relevant problem in urgent need of innovative, alternative management approaches targeting underlying mechanisms.

Regarding mechanisms, the central discovery in pain research over the last quarter century is that noxious input results in altered pain processing, particularly central, and that such alterations are also seen in the context of developing and established chronic pain. It thus appears logical to conclude that making altered pain processing visible in patients in the clinical context – and then targeting these alterations therapeutically – may be key in achieving effective mechanism-orientated management of the hitherto intractable problem of chronic pain and its development.

The work presented here is the result of almost two decades of clinical research using quantitative sensory testing (QST), an accepted – but hitherto mainly experimental – tool for revealing altered somatosensory processing. The outcome of my research programme is a new, systematic, mechanism-orientated approach for the successful management of chronic pain and its genesis in everyday clinical practice.

The *first* major thrust of my research programme was to set up and validate a screening QST paradigm, the **N**ijmegen-**A**alborg **S**creening **Q**ST (**NASQ**) paradigm, designed for systematic diagnosis of altered central pain processing in clinical pain patients. The main characteristics of the NASQ paradigm are as follows:

- it is suitable and validated for use in clinical pain patients, lasting about 30 minutes
- it reveals the topography of altered pain processing via skin and deep tissue stimuli

- it contains both static (pain sensitivity) and dynamic (pain modulation) elements
- it diagnoses central sensitisation and pro-nociceptive shifts in pain modulation

The *second* major thrust of my research was to systematically implement and validate NASQ in clinical pain practice. This I did by developing a **S**ystematic **A**pproach **T**o **A**ltered **P**ain **P**rocessing using **QST** (**SATAPP.QST**) as the basis for a paradigm shift towards mechanism-orientated approaches to pain disease diagnosis and treatment. SATAPP.QST provides this basis by answering four key questions about altered pain processing in pain disorders:

- What is the source of nociception?
- Is nociceptive transmission altered?
- Is central pain processing altered?
- Is altered central processing dependent on peripheral nociceptive drive?

The *first* area to which I applied SATAPP.QST was in *perioperative patients*. Pain is a major negative outcome after surgery; its prevention and treatment represents a major clinical challenge. Using NASQ I have achieved the first systematic documentation of altered perioperative pain processing by measuring pain sensitivity at multiple sites, for skin and muscle, preoperatively and short-term (first week) and long-term (for six months) after surgery. I also measured descending pain modulation via conditioned pain modulation (CPM) paradigm using a cold pressor task.

The perioperative application of NASQ has permitted me to provide the first and only comprehensive description available to date of neuroplasticity after surgery and the factors influencing it. The first week after surgery, after an initial 24 hour inhibitory phase, augmented pain sensitivity becomes increasingly manifest. This hyperalgesia spreads rapidly away from the site of surgery and is more pronounced in the absence of adequate analgesia during surgery and in vulnerable patients (i.e. preoperative pain, nerve damage). Patients reporting chronic pain six months after surgery consistently manifest more spreading hyperalgesia throughout the preceding six months, both of skin and muscle. Greater vulnerability to spreading hyperalgesia – and to chronic pain – correlates with weaker preoperative descending inhibitory pain modulation.

Chronic pain development after surgery is thus associated with persistence and rostral spread of neuraxial central sensitisation, a process facilitated by preoperative pro-nociceptive shifts in descending pain modulation. SATAPP.QST for the first time makes it possible to achieve rational and effective perioperative pain management by enabling: 1) preoperative assessment for risk of chronic pain after surgery, 2) postoperative monitoring for early signs of chronic pain development, and 3) monitoring of effectiveness of perioperative management regarding chronic pain prevention and treatment.

The *second area* in which I investigated SATAPP.QST was in the diagnosis and management of four intractable *chronic pain conditions* of different aetiologies. Using the NASQ paradigm we studied patients with 1) complex regional pain syndrome (CRPS) type I (neuroinflammatory pain), 2) chronic low back pain (somatic and neuropathic pain), 3) chronic pancreatitis (viscero-somatic pain), and 4) dysmenorrhoea (viscero-visceral pain). My key finding was that chronic pain disorders are consistently linked to spreading, heterotopic deep tissue hyperalgesia – regardless of the original diagnosis. This ground-breaking finding is congruent with my studies on pain persistence after surgery, and indicates that persistent, rostrally spreading central sensitisation is key to chronic pain and its development.

Clinical application of NASQ has resulted in pioneering conclusions central to achieving SATAPP.QST-based management of chronic pain. The first-ever clinical implementation of such an approach by my group has revolutionised our own pain practice. The innovative findings resulting from my research on chronic pain may be summarised as follows:

- Spreading, heterotopic deep tissue hyperalgesia is diagnostic for chronic pain,
- Hyperalgesia spread differs with disease subtype, and is linked to pain progression,
- Central sensitisation manifest as spreading hyperalgesia can become independent of peripheral nociceptive inputs, thus no longer responding to peripheral deafferentation treatments, e.g. nerve blocks, opioids,
- Specific targeted treatments, e.g. the NMDA antagonist S-ketamine, are necessary to inhibit central sensitisation manifest as spreading hyperalgesia,
- Clinical pain measures and QST measures correlate poorly, thus QST and clinical pain measures yield different but complementary information.

Application of SATAPP.QST in clinical chronic pain practice thus permits a key paradigm shift towards mechanism-orientated management by enabling: 1) diagnosis and prognosis of chronic pain, including subtype definition, 2) monitoring for signs of chronic pain progression, 3) rational treatment choices for maximal treatment response, and 4) ongoing monitoring of effectiveness of chronic pain management.

In conclusion, altered central pain processing is key to understanding the mechanisms of chronic pain and its genesis. QST methods are necessary to reliably diagnose alterations in pain processing. My research programme for the first time provides a comprehensive and practical basis for the urgently needed paradigm shift in pain medicine away from symptom-based management towards a mechanism-orientated approach to altered pain processing. ***This shift can be implemented in clinical practice now***, based on the systematic framework (SATAPP.QST) and accompanying tools (NASQ) validated by my research. My studies show that NASQ makes visible altered pain processing and represents a valid clinical diagnostic method, and that SATAPP.QST implementation provides real clinical benefit in the diagnostics, prognostics and monitoring of chronic pain disorders and their progression. Furthermore, we provide first evidence that pain management paradigms based on SATAPP.QST are feasible and successful when implemented in clinical practice.

Danish Summary (Sammenfatning)

Vedvarende smerter efter heling af væv, som har været udsat for traume, samt efterfølgende kroniske smertesyndromer har store personlige og samfundsmæssige omkostninger. På trods af de seneste årtiers intense og koordinerede indsats for at opnå effektiv behandling ved hjælp af videnskabelige og organisatoriske fremskridt er der kun fremkommet små reelle forbedringer med den nuværende symptombaserede terapeutiske tilgang til imødegåelse og behandling af kroniske smerter. Kroniske smerter og udviklingen heraf er derfor stadig et stort klinisk relevant problem, som kræver innovative og alternative behandlingstilgange, som målrettes mod de underliggende mekanismer.

Med hensyn til mekanismerne er den centrale opdagelse inden for smerteforskningen i de seneste 25 år, at giftige input resulterer i ændret smertebearbejdning, især centralt, og at sådanne ændringer også ses i sammenhæng med udvikling og etablering af kronisk smerte. Det synes derfor logisk at konkludere, at en tydeliggørelse af den ændrede smertebearbejdning hos patienter i klinisk sammenhæng – efterfulgt af en målrettet terapeutisk indsats mod disse ændringer – kan være nøglen til at opnå en effektiv mekanismeorienteret håndtering af det hidtil intraktable problem med kroniske smerter og deres udvikling.

Det arbejde, som præsenteres her, er resultatet af næsten to årtiers klinisk forskning ved hjælp af kvantitative sensoriske tests (QST), som er et anerkendt – men hidtil mest eksperimentelt anvendt – værktøj til påvisning af ændret somatosensorisk bearbejdelse. Resultatet af mit forskningsprogram er en ny, systematisk mekanisme-orienteret tilgang, som sikrer succesfuld behandling af kronisk smerte i klinisk praksis samt viden om, hvorfor smerten opstår.

Den *første* betydelige del af mit forskningsprogram bestod i at opsætte og validere et screenings-QST paradigme (The **N**ijmegen-**A**alborg **S**creening **Q**ST (**NASQ**) Paradigm) for systematisk diagnosticering af ændret central smertebearbejdning hos kliniske smertepatienter. NASQ-paradigmet kendes på følgende:

- det er velegnet og valideret til brug på kliniske patienter (varighed ca. 30 minutter)
- det afdækker topografien af ændret smertebearbejdning ved hjælp af stimuli på hud og i dybe væv
- det indeholder både statiske (smertefølsomhed) og dynamiske (smerte-modulation) elementer
- det diagnosticerer central sensibilisering og pro-nociceptive ændringer i smertemodulationen

Den *anden* store del af mit forskningsprogram bestod i en systematisk implementering og validering af NASQ i klinisk praksis. Til dette formål udviklede jeg metoden "en systematisk tilgang til ændret smertebearbejdning ved hjælp af QST" (A **S**ystematic **A**pproach **T**o **A**ltered **P**ain **P**rocessing using **QST** (**SATAPP.QST**)) som grundlag for et paradigmeskifte mod mere mekanisme-orienterede tilgange til diagnosticering og behandling af smertelidelser. SATAPP.QST danner grundlag for besvarelse af fire hovedspørgsmål om den ændrede smertebearbejdning hos patienter med smertelidelser:

- Hvad er kilden til nociception?
- Ændres den nociceptive transmission?
- Ændres den centrale smertebearbejdning?
- Er ændret central bearbejdning afhængig a perifert nociceptiv drive?

Den *første* gruppe, hvorpå SATAPP.QST blev anvendt, var *perioperative patienter.* Smerter er et væsentligt negativt resultat af operationer; forhindring og behandling af smerter udgør derfor en stor klinisk udfordring. Ved hjælp af NASQ har jeg opnået den første systematiske dokumentation af ændret perioperativ smertebearbejdning ved at måle smertefølsomheden flere steder (på hud og i muskler) før operation, kort efter (efter en uge) og lang tid efter operation (efter seks måneder). Jeg målte også den descenderende smertemodulation ved hjælp af et paradigme for konditioneret smertemodulation (CPM) indeholdende en kold pressor test.

Den perioperative anvendelse af NASQ har gjort det muligt for mig at udarbejde den første, hidtil eneste og mest omfattende beskrivelse af neuro-plasticitet efter operation samt de faktorer, der påvirker denne. Den første uge efter operationen, efter en indledende 24-timers hæmmende fase, manifesteres en forstærket smertefølsomhed. Denne hyperalgesi spredes hurtigt væk fra operationsstedet og bliver mere udtalt i tilfælde med utilstrækkelig bedøvelse under operationen og hos sårbare patienter (dvs. patienter med præoperative smerter eller med nerveskader). Patienter, der rapporterer om kroniske smerter et halvt år efter en operation, udviser konsekvent mere spredt hyperalgesi i de seks måneder både i hud og muskler. Større sårbarhed over for udbredt hyperalgesi – og over for kronisk smerte – korrelerer med svagere præoperativ descenderende hæmmende smertemodulation.

Udvikling af kronisk smerte efter operation forbindes derfor med vedholdenhed og rostral spredning af neuraxial central sensibilisering; en proces, som faciliteres af præoperative pro-nociceptive ændringer i den descenderende smertemodulation. SATAPP.QST gør det for første gang muligt at udføre en rationel og effektiv perioperativ smertehåndtering ved hjælp af: 1) en præoperativ vurdering af risikoen for kronisk smerte efter operation, 2) en postoperativ monitorering af tidlige tegn på udvikling af kronisk smerte og 3) monitorering af effektiviteten af den perioperative håndtering med hensyn til opstået og behandling af kronisk smerte.

Det andet *område*, hvor jeg undersøgte SATAPP.QST, var i forbindelse med diagnose og behandling af fire intraktable kroniske smertelidelser med forskellig ætiologi. Ved hjælp af NASQ-paradigmet undersøgte vi patienter med 1) komplekst regionalt smertesyndrom (CRPS) type 1 (neuro-inflam matorisk smerte), 2) kroniske lændesmerter (somatisk og neuropatisk smerte), 3) kronisk pankreatitis (viscero-somatisk smerte) og 4) dysmenoré (visceroviscerale smerte). Det vigtigste resultat var, at kroniske smertelidelser konsekvent er forbundet med spredt heterotopisk hyperalgesi i dybt væv – uanset hvilken diagnose, der oprindeligt var stillet. Dette banebrydende resultat er i overensstemmelse med mine studier i vedvarende smerter efter operation og indikerer, at vedvarende rostral spredt central sensibilisering er nøglen til kronisk smerte og udviklingen heraf.

Den kliniske anvendelse af NASQ har resulteret i banebrydende konklusioner, som er centrale for at kunne udføre en SATAPP.QST-baseret håndtering af kronisk smerte. Min forskningsgruppe har som de første implementeret denne fremgangsmåde, hvilket har revolutioneret vores smertepraksis. De nyskabende resultater af min forskning i kronisk smerte kan opsummeres som følger:

- Spredt heterotopisk hyperalgesi i dybt væv er diagnosen for kronisk smerte
- Spredningen af hyperalgesi varierer afhængig af lidelsens type og er forbundet med smerteudvikling
- Central sensibilisering - manifesteret som spredt hyperalgesi - kan blive uafhængig af perifere nociceptive input og reagerer således ikke længere på perifere deafferentationsbehandlinger, f.eks. nerveblokader og opioider

- Specifikke målrettede behandlinger, f.eks. NMDA antagonist S-ketamin, er nødvendige for at inhibere central sensibilisering manifesteret som spredt hyperalgesi
- Kliniske smertemål og QST-målinger korrelerer dårligt, således at QST og kliniske smertemålinger giver forskellig men komplementær information

Anvendelse af SATAPP.QST i klinisk praksis på kroniske smerter tillader således et paradigmeskifte mod en mere mekanisme-orienteret behandling, som gør det muligt, 1) at diagnosticere og opstille en prognose for kronisk smerte inklusive definition af undertype, 2) at monitorere tegn på udvikling af kronisk smerte, 3) at træffe rationelle behandlingsvalg for opnåelse af det bedst mulige behandlingsrespons og 4) at udføre løbende monitorering af effektiviteten af håndteringen af den kroniske smerte.

Afslutningsvis skal det nævnes, at ændret central smertebearbejdning er nøglen til at forstå mekanismerne i kronisk smerte og dens opståen. QST-metoderne er nødvendige for at kunne stille en sikker diagnose vedrørende ændringer i smertebearbejdningen. Min forskning har skabt det første omfattende og praktiske grundlag for et presserende paradigmeskifte inden for smertemedicin; væk fra den symptombaserede behandling og mod en mekanismeorienteret tilgang til den ændrede smertebearbejdning. *Det er nu muligt at implementere skiftet i klinisk praksis* baseret på det systematiske grundlag (SATAPP.QST) med det tilhørende værktøj (NASQ), som min forskning har valideret. Mine studier viser, at NASQ synliggør en ændret smertebearbejdning og repræsenterer en valid klinisk diagnosticeringsmetode samt at implementering af SATAPP.QST giver reelle kliniske fordele inden for diagnosticering, prognostik og monitorering af kroniske smertelidelser og deres udvikling. Endvidere har vi fremlagt de første beviser på, at smertehåndteringsparadigmer baseret på SATAPP.QST er praktiserbare og succesfulde, når de implementeres i klinisk praksis.

Dissertation Articles

1. Wilder-Smith OH, Tassonyi E, Senly C, Otten P, Arendt-Nielsen L. Surgical pain is followed not only by spinal sensitization but also by supraspinal antinociception. Br J Anaesth. 1996 Jun;76,(6):816–21. (I)
2. Wilder-Smith OH, Arendt-Nielsen L, Gäumann D, Tassonyi E, Rifat KR. Sensory changes and pain after abdominal hysterectomy: a comparison of anesthetic supplementation with fentanyl versus magnesium or ketamine. Anesth Analg. 1998 Jan;86(1):95–101. (II)
3. Wilder-Smith OH, Möhrle JJ, Dolin PJ, Martin NC. The management of chronic pain in Switzerland: a comparative survey of Swiss medical specialists treating chronic pain. Eur J Pain. 2001;5(3):285–98. (III)
4. Wilder-Smith OH, Möhrle JJ, Martin NC. Acute pain management after surgery or in the emergency room in Switzerland: a comparative survey of Swiss anaesthesiologists and surgeons. Eur J Pain. 2002;6(3):189–201. (IV)
5. Wilder-Smith OH, Tassonyi E, Arendt-Nielsen L. Preoperative back pain is associated with diverse manifestations of central neuroplasticity. Pain. 2002 Jun;97(3):189–94. (V)
6. Wilder-Smith OH, Tassonyi E, Crul BJ, Arendt-Nielsen L. Quantitative sensory testing and human surgery: effects of analgesic management on postoperative neuroplasticity. Anesthesiology. 2003 May;98(5):1214–22. (VI)
7. Vaneker M, Wilder-Smith OH, Schrombges P, de Man-Hermsen I, Oerlemans HM. Patients initially diagnosed as 'warm' or 'cold' CRPS 1 show differences in central sensory processing some eight years after diagnosis: a quantitative sensory testing study. Pain. 2005 May;115(1–2):204–11. (VII)
8. Buscher HC, Wilder-Smith OH, van Goor H. Chronic pancreatitis patients show hyperalgesia of central origin: a pilot study. Eur J Pain. 2006 May;10(4):363–70. (VIII)
9. Buscher HC, van Goor H, Wilder-Smith OH. Effect of thoracoscopic splanchnic denervation on pain processing in chronic pancreatitis patients. Eur J Pain. 2007 May;11(4):437–43. (IX)

10. Brinkert W, Dimcevski G, Arendt-Nielsen L, Drewes AM, Wilder-Smith OH. Dysmenorrhoea is associated with hypersensitivity in the sigmoid colon and rectum. Pain. 2007 Nov;132 Suppl 1:S46–51. (X)
11. Steegers MA, Wolters B, Evers AW, Strobbe L, Wilder-Smith OH. Effect of axillary lymph node dissection on prevalence and intensity of chronic and phantom pain after breast cancer surgery. J Pain. 2008 Sep;9(9): 813–22. (XI)
12. Steegers MA, Snik DM, Verhagen AF, van der Drift MA, Wilder-Smith OH. Only half of the chronic pain after thoracic surgery shows a neuropathic component. J Pain. 2008 Oct;9(10):955–61. (XII)
13. Wilder-Smith OH, Schreyer T, Scheffer GJ, Arendt-Nielsen L. Patients with chronic pain after abdominal surgery show less preoperative endogenous pain inhibition and more postoperative hyperalgesia: a pilot study. J Pain Palliat Care Pharmacother. 2010 Jun;24(2):119–28. (XIII)
14. Bouwense SA, Buscher HC, van Goor H, Wilder-Smith OH. S-ketamine modulates hyperalgesia in patients with chronic pancreatitis pain. Reg Anesth Pain Med. 2011 May-Jun;36(3):303–7. (XIV)
15. Bouwense SA, Buscher HC, van Goor H, Wilder-Smith OH. Has central sensitization become independent of nociceptive input in chronic pancreatitis patients who fail thoracoscopic splanchnicectomy? Reg Anesth Pain Med. 2011 Nov-Dec;36(6):531–6. (XV)

1

Introduction

Pain, both acute and chronic, is an unpleasant but common part of life. In its acute form, it carries an important warning message to the person suffering from it, namely to change his behaviour to avoid further harm and damage. However, in some patients, pain does not go away after the acute episode, and persists, losing its useful warning message connected to the avoidance of tissue damage. Ultimately it becomes chronic pain, a disease of pain processing in its own right.

How this transition from a useful adaptive physiological response to a maladaptive pathological process occurs, the nature of this maladaptive response, and how it progresses over time has been a central question of pain research for the last few decades. My particular interest in this field – and the subject of my research for the last fifteen years – has been, *firstly*, how to effectively diagnose such chronic pain in patients, particularly its genesis and its progression, and, *secondly*, by the clinical implementation of such diagnostics to lay the foundation for successful chronic pain management in daily practice.

1.1 Defining the Problem

1.1.1 Acute Pain

Acute pain is the pain accompanying some form of tissue damage or trauma, and is usually considered to last a few days after the event. A much-studied model of acute pain is that accompanying surgery. Typically surgery is accompanied by severe acute pain in the first few days after surgery, with pain being spontaneous, ongoing or evoked by movement (coughing, mobilisation). The pain is usually most severe the first and second days after surgery, gradually decreasing thereafter to usually disappear – at least in its spontaneous or ongoing form – at the end of the first postoperative week[1,2].

In a recent study of major surgical interventions 43%, 27% and 16% of patients experienced significant spontaneous or ongoing pain (VAS $\geq$ 40 mm) on postoperative days 1, 2 and 3, respectively 2. For any type of pain – ongoing or evoked – the respective incidences of significant pain (VAS $\geq$ 40 mm) for postoperative days 1, 2 and 3 were 88%, 81% and 72%[2]. In reviewing the literature, major postoperative pain appears to be present in between 30 – 70% of surgical patients, with at least 20% achieving inadequate pain relief overall[3,4]. Unfortunately, it has to be noted that acute postoperative pain management has not improved over the last decade despite a variety of concerted attempts at improvement during this period[4,5].

1.1.2 Persistent Postoperative Pain

Pain persisting beyond three to five days after surgery is only now being recognised as a negative outcome in its own right. Thirty to fifty percent of patients undergoing amputation, mastectomy, thoracotomy or sternotomy still show persistent pain 3–6 months after surgery, with 5 – 10% of these reporting severe pain[6-8]. Even "minor" interventions such as inguinal herniorrhaphy are associated with significant incidences of postoperative persistent pain 9. Approx. one third of inguinal herniorrhaphy patients still complain of moderate or severe pain one week after surgery, with the figure at one month and one year being 10% and 10–15%, respectively[9-11]. If we combine the many operations performed each year (NL: more than 1.5 million) with the acute and persistent pain incidences just cited, pain after surgery has a major and significant medical and societal impact. It should be noted that once persistent pain becomes chronic pain, a maximum of one third of the patients will benefit from presently available therapeutic options[6,8].

1.1.3 Chronic Pain

Established chronic pain is defined by the International Association for the Study of Pain (IASP) as pain present for longer than six months. Chronic pain, not only of surgical but also of non-surgical origin, is a major medical and societal problem in the Western world. Chronic widespread musculoskeletal pain, for example, is reported in ca. 10% of the general population[12]. In 1995, total Dutch costs for low back pain, the commonest form of chronic pain, were estimated at some EUR 3.7 billion per year, equivalent to almost 2% of the gross national product and a per capita cost per year of EUR 240[13]. In a large Dutch general population study, almost half the respondents had low back pain in the past year, and some 40% reported that the episode was continuously present or had lasted more than 12 weeks[14]. 62% of low back pain sufferers still have pain 12 months later, with acute recurrence within one year of an episode in up to 73%, and a lifetime recurrence rate of up to 85%[15−17]. Over 90% of low back pain costs are indirect and related to work and invalidity, with a small group of patients (10–25%) with recurrent, long-lasting and severe low back pain causing 75% of total costs[13,18,19]. Thus limited treatment success and major societal impact define presently practised conservative as well as the interventional low back pain management options[17,19−23]. Again it should be noted that also in the field of chronic pain, there is an ample body of research identifying the limited impact of current standard therapeutic approaches.

1.1.4 Summary

In summary, chronic pain and the transition from acute to chronic pain continues to have a major societal impact regarding suffering and cost. Despite major and concerted efforts in the last two decades at achieving effective management of this problem through scientific and organisational advances, little real impression has been made by present therapeutic approaches on the prevention and treatment of chronic pain. Thus chronic pain must be regarded as a frequent, clinically relevant and undesirable societal and medical problem in urgent need of new, effective management approaches.

1.2 The Key: Pain and Neuroplasticity

In contrast to the ongoing practical problems in achieving a clinical therapeutic impact on pain, fundamental research regarding pain and its underlying mechanisms has been more successful. Thus the last two decades have seen crucial and significant improvements in our understanding of the mechanisms underlying nociception and pain. A key insight has been that nervous system processing of nociception and pain is not hard-wired, and that the gain of the nervous system typically changes as a result of noxious sensory inputs. Acute nociception typically initially results in increased pain sensitivity (hyperalgesia) affecting the peripheral and central nervous system[24−26]. Initially, it sensitises the peripheral nervous system via excitatory substance release from damaged tissues and nerves. The resulting nociceptive barrage to spinal cord, brainstem and brain in turn excites the central nervous system (central sensitisation), further increasing sensitivity.

1.2.1 Excitatory Neuroplasticity

In basic animal models, excitatory neuroplasticity (i.e. "sensitisation") moves from activation (acute, transient, activity-dependent) via modulation (sub-acute, slower, but still reversible functional changes) through to modification (chronic structural and architectural alterations)[25]. Activation involves use-dependent augmentation of transduction (peripheral nociceptors, autosensitisation) and transmission (central processing, wind-up) and should be considered a rapidly reversible physiological process[25]. Modulation expresses itself in peripheral and central sensitisation, mainly due to phosphorylation of neuronal receptors and ionophores; it is a more slowly reversible process with early pathological connotations[25]. Modification is considered the basis of chronic, pathological pain, and entails altered regulation and cell connectivity together with cell death, particularly affecting inhibitory systems[25].

1.2.2 Inhibitory Neuroplasticity

For intact organisms, these excitatory changes quickly elicit counteracting inhibitory responses[27]. Such inhibitory responses, an integral part of the complex modulation excitatory nociceptive transmission normally undergoes from peripheral to central in the nervous system[28,29], can be spinal or supraspinal. The latter, also termed descending inhibition, operates via multiple tonic and phasic systems, originates in medulla and midbrain, and is closely related to parallel descending facilitatory systems[28-31]. The ability to produce an inhibitory response (e.g. diffuse noxious inhibitory controls, DNIC) is now considered to be an important prognostic factor for human development of chronic pain, and its absence may contribute to increase the initial excitatory responses described above[32,33]. The quality of inhibitory responses may carry important prognostic information regarding susceptibility to chronic pain[33-35].

1.2.3 Clinical Reality of Neuroplasticity

The reality of the changes in sensory processing accompanying human acute pain, e.g. due to surgery, is now well demonstrated, both by my research (I, II, IV, VIII, IX, X) and by other groups[36-42]. Sensitised pain processing and pro-nociceptive pain modulation have further been demonstrated to accompany and characterise many human chronic pain diseases[43], including low back pain (III)[44,45], fibromyalgia[46-48], osteoarthritis[32], CRPS (VII)[49] and visceral pain (VI,VII, X)[50]. Furthermore, in large cross-sectional population studies, it has been demonstrated that more pro-nociceptive pain processing (e.g. poorer DNIC) is also associated with a greater risk of chronic pain in general[33,35].

1.2.4 Summary

In summary, the key finding of pain research of the last decades has been that nociceptive input results in altered pain processing, and that such alterations in pain processing are also seen in the context of developing and established chronic pain. From these findings, it appears logical to conclude that making such alterations in pain processing visible in patients in the clinical context – and then targeting these therapeutically – may be the key to achieving effective management approaches to the hitherto largely intractable problem of chronic pain and its development.

1.3 The Tool: Quantitative Sensory Processing (QST)

Over the last couple of decades quantitative sensory testing (QST), also termed psychophysical testing, has emerged as a potential tool for monitoring and diagnosing pain processing and its alterations in patients[51–54]. This technique is based on the application of defined stimuli to the patient under standardized conditions, and then asking the patient to rate the stimulus regarding its experienced intensity. The use of multiple stimuli with differing intensities makes it possible to construct stimulus-response relationships characterizing the state of the patient's pain processing (Figure 1).

This technique has the advantage of permitting assessment of the entire pain stimulus-response curve from subthreshold to suprathreshold input. The major disadvantage of this approach is that it is time-consuming, and requires that the subject be well trained in rating pain stimuli accurately and reliably [55].

In clinical practice, the procedure is often simplified by determining only one point on the stimulus-response curve, namely a threshold for the transition to pain (the pain threshold) or "intolerable" pain (the pain tolerance threshold). Thresholds are typically determined using a simple ramping procedure, which is quick, but subject to anticipation effects and reaction time (Figure 2,). Up-and-down techniques such as the method of limits are more accurate, with the disadvantage of being more time-consuming (Figure 3, below)[52,55,56]. Thresholds are a frequently used monoparameter for clinical research into pain processing as it is quick and easy to train patients in their use. The limitations

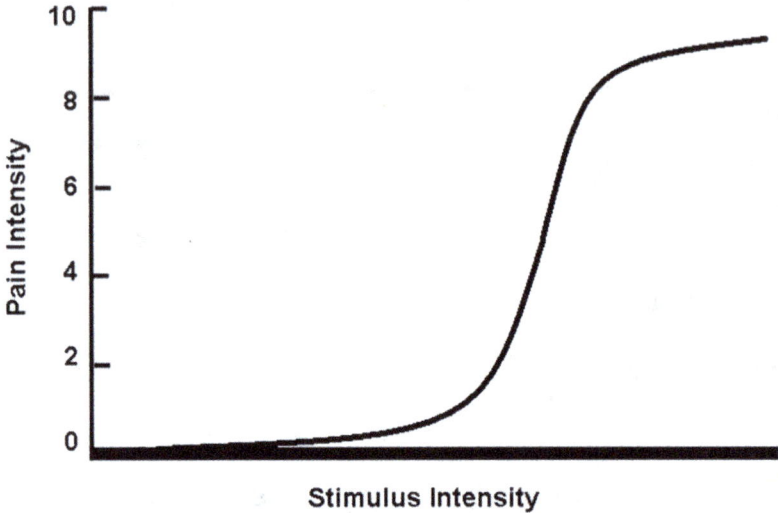

Figure 1   Typical stimulus-response curve obtained from plotting responses obtained from multiple stimuli during quantitative sensory testing

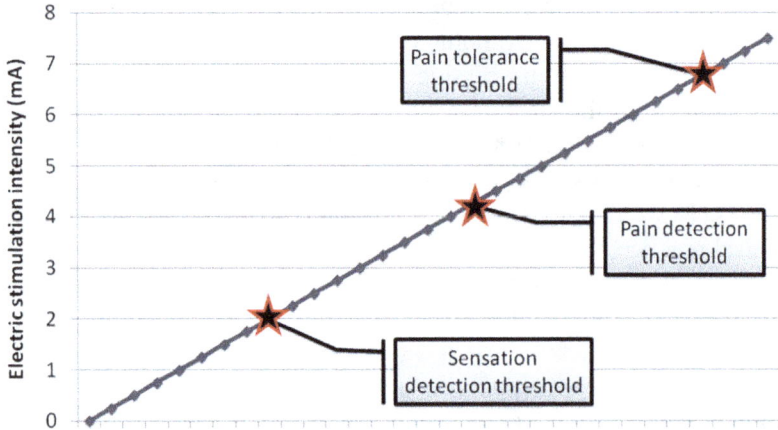

Figure 2   Ramping quantitative sensory testing involving application of stimuli of increasing intensity. Here, multiple thresholds can be determined, e.g. sensation or pain detection threshold or pain tolerance threshold

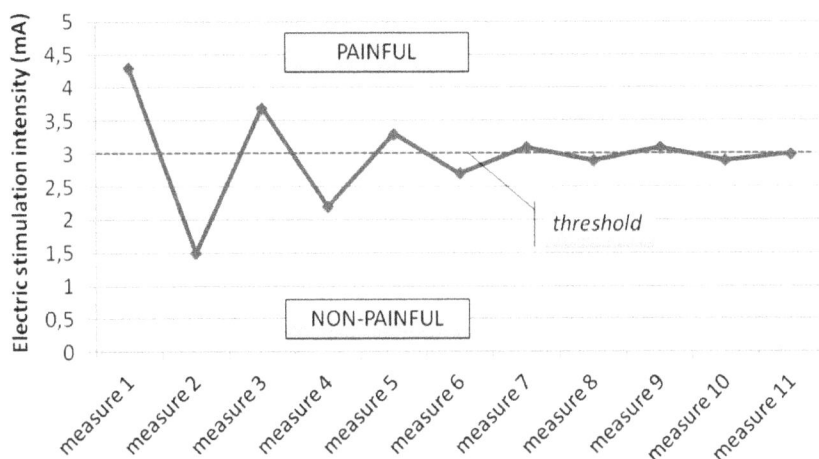

Figure 3 Method of limits approach, involving successive stimuli above and below threshold gradually closing down on the pain threshold

of such a monoparameter, particularly if it does not involve suprathreshold stimulation, must, however, be kept in mind when interpreting it as a measure of pain processing.

The information derived from QST about pain processing can be increased by stimulation of different tissues (e.g. skin, muscle, viscera) in a variety of anatomical locations (topography, e.g. to distinguish between segmental and generalized hyperalgesia). Further information can be obtained by altering the nature of the stimulus (e.g. thermal, mechanical, electrical, chemical), or by investigating the effect of a conditioning stimulus (e.g. a cold pressor task via ice water bucket immersion) on pain processing by applying test stimulation before, during and after conditioning stimulation. A typical example of the latter is the diffuse noxious inhibitory controls (DNIC) paradigm[32,57–61,] also called a conditioned pain modulation (CPM) paradigm[62–66]. The CPM (or DNIC) paradigm (Figure 4, below) is robust and relatively insensitive to minor details of experimental setup, and makes it possible to visualize the effectiveness of phasic descending inhibitory mechanisms – or the pro- vs. antinociceptive balance – in a given patient or patient population[33,34,60,61,66].

In summary, QST techniques are potentially useful in diagnosing a variety of aspects of the pain processing state of patients. QST can be either static (test stimuli only) or dynamic (test and conditioning stimuli), with the former providing information about basal pain sensitivity, while the latter provides information about pain modulation. The results can be interpreted either at

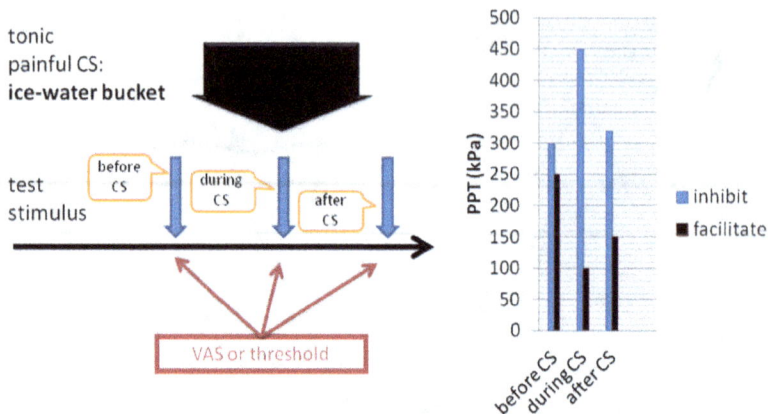

Figure 4   Conditioned pain modulation (CPM) paradigm for testing descending modulation of pain inputs. The effect of a tonic painful conditioning stimulus (CS) is revealed by test stimuli applied before, during and after conditioning stimulation. Test stimuli are quantified either by determining pain experience (e.g. pain VAS) or pain thresholds (e.g. pressure pain threshold (PPT) in kPa). Graph on right shows PPTs before, during and after conditioning stimulus with either inhibitory (inhibit) or facilitatory (facilitate) modulation

a given time in reference to normal value data (e.g.[67,68]), or in the context of disease progression via multiple measures in time. We have demonstrated the latter approach is particularly valuable in the perioperative context, as many patients are pain-free before surgery and can therefore serve as their own normal controls (I, II, VI, XIII).

1.4 The Solution: A Systematic Approach to Altered Pain Processing (SATAPP)

Why have we been so unsuccessful in improving outcomes of human pain diseases despite the impressive advances in animal experimental understanding of pain mechanisms summarised above? I consider three related reasons to underlie this problem, which will be discussed in the following sections.

1.4.1 Translation Difficulties

The *first reason* has to do with the basal scientific knowledge which our practice of pain medicine is based upon, and the difficulties of translating the results of animal research to human clinical practice. As already discussed, basic animal research has certainly been successful in unravelling the mechanisms underlying various aspects of pain – in animals. However, difficulties arise when one attempts to extrapolate findings from animal research directly to the human situation. A major reason is the different endpoints which are used in animals and patient pain research. Resolution of this problem requires a determined effort to use the same endpoints reflecting similar mechanisms in animal and human research. One candidate for achieving this goal is the use of measures reflecting alterations in pain processing common to both animal and humans. It should be noted that this approach can be complicated by the differences in the anatomy and physiology of pain processing in animals vs. humans, particularly regarding more rostral neuraxial (e.g. cortical) aspects of pain processing important in chronic pain and its development[69,70].

The practical consequences of translational problems are illustrated by the pre-emptive analgesia debate[71–74], and the ongoing difficulties in the use of animal models for the development of analgesic drugs for clinical human use[75]. In both cases, predictions regarding clinical treatment approaches based on pain mechanisms elucidated in animal models fail to be accurate in the human clinical context, resulting in lack of success of the derived therapeutic concepts. The main reason for this failure was that different endpoints were used in animals and humans, namely altered pain processing in animals, versus altered pain experience in humans[27].

1.4.2 Symptoms vs. Altered Pain Processing

The *second reason* is that current clinical pain treatment continues to be essentially symptom-based, palliating symptoms instead of targeting underlying alterations in pain processing[76]. As detailed above, we have come to the point of being forced to accept that there is a limit to what can be achieved therapeutically with our present empirical, symptom-based approach to pain, particularly regarding chronic pain and its development[8,17, 19–23,27]. This finding is only reinforced by recent unsuccessful attempts to derive insights into possible underlying mechanisms from a systematised approach to clinical physical signs of pain disorders[77]. In fact, a recent fMRI study of chronic low back pain patients comments that changes in brain pain processing explain 70–80% of pain variance, as opposed to the 20–25% explained by traditional biopsychosocial factors upon which symptom-based treatment is based[21,78]. What is thus necessary is a major shift of emphasis away from symptoms of pain experience and towards the alterations in pain processing underlying pain disorders.

1.4.3 Documenting Altered Pain Processing in Human Pain Patients

This necessary shift in emphasis brings us to the *third reason*, namely that the work of systematically and comprehensively understanding the pathophysiological processes and mechanisms active on a systems level in the nervous system *of actual human pain patients* has barely begun. These necessary insights into diseased pain processing mechanisms can never be generated with adequate certainty or detail from animal or human healthy volunteer research: they must be collected from actual human pain patients in the clinical context. Although this approach may appear onerous, the advantage of it is that, once realised, it also permits rapid clinical application of the knowledge and technology so generated. Systematic application of the knowledge concerning altered pain processing provided by such clinical research is the basis for achieving effective treatment for chronic pain and its development orientated towards altered pain processing – rather than based on pain symptoms. Key in this context is the implementation in everyday clinical practice of the diagnostic technologies developed in the course of research targeting altered pain processing.

1.4.4 The Challenge: Achieving a Systematic Approach to Altered Pain Processing in Patients

In summary, it is time to institute a fundamental paradigm shift in clinical pain medicine. This shift requires that we leave behind old empirical symptom-based methods and move towards a new, ***systematic approach to altered pain processing (SATAPP)*** in pain disorders. Achieving this paradigm shifting approach requires concerted research and development activities in three areas, namely:

1) Development of diagnostic techniques informing about altered pain processing in the human clinical context,
2) Use of these diagnostic techniques to define the alterations in pain processing typically accompanying human pain disorders, and
3) Identification and development of a comprehensive therapeutic armamentarium targeting various aspects of altered pain processing.

Based upon research and development in these three areas, we can achieve the development and validation of a comprehensive systematic approach to altered pain processing based on QST (SATAPP.QST) as the foundation for successful diagnostics and therapeutics of human pain disorders.

1.5 Aim of the Present Review: Implementing SATAPP.QST in Pain Medicine

The aim of the present review is to provide a basis for the just-described paradigm shift in pain medicine away from symptom-based management towards a systematic approach to altered pain processing in pain diseases. Based on the research I have done over the last fifteen years, the review will concentrate on demonstrating the following:

1) Quantitative sensory testing (QST) represents a valid method of diagnostics for altered pain processing now suitable for implementation into routine clinical practice;

2) Implementation of diagnostics targeting altered pain processing using QST provides real clinical benefit in the diagnostics, prognostics and monitoring of chronic pain disorders and their progression;

3) First examples of pain management paradigms effectively targeting altered pain processing are now available, without going into pharmacological details of specific drug regimes, which lie beyond the scope of the present work; and

4) Based on 1–3, achieving and implementing a systematic approach to altered pain processing based on QST (SATAPP.QST) regarding pain diagnostics and therapeutics in clinical pain practice is now feasible.

2

SATAPP.QST

2.1 Clinical Application of SATAPP in Pain Disorders

To achieve the paradigm shift towards a systematic approach to altered pain processing (SATAPP) in pain medicine discussed above, I consider it essential to provide answers to the following **four key diagnostic questions** regarding pain disorders in the clinical context:

2.1.1 What is the Peripheral Source of Nociceptive Input?

We assume that most chronic pain disorders start off with a nociceptive source. Knowledge of this source and its nature enables us to try to deal therapeutically with the source, or to try deafferenting it with drugs or invasive procedures. Furthermore, this information permits identification of particularly aggressive types of nociceptive input (e.g. visceral pain).

2.1.2 Is Nociceptive Transmission from Periphery to Centre Altered?

Nerve damage is a common reason for altered nociceptive transmission from periphery to centre. Diagnosis of nerve damage is particularly important because it is a strong predisposing factor to aggressive alterations in central pain processing. Furthermore, damaged nerves can in themselves be an additional source of aggressive nociceptive input.

2.1.3 Is Central Nociceptive Processing Altered?

Answering this question is central to achieving SATAPP, and quantitative sensory testing (QST) is the key to diagnosing altered central nociceptive processing. Two main classes of altered central pain processing are described in the literature, necessitating the following two basic questions:

Firstly: has central sensitivity to pain altered? The presence and persistence of central sensitisation has significant prognostic and therapeutic

13

consequences, as previously discussed. More extensive spread of central sensitisation can indicate more advanced or serious pain disease. Furthermore, the presence of central sensitisation makes measures aiming at peripheral deafferentation less effective, and requires the use of own specific and targeted therapeutic approaches.

Secondly: what is the state of descending central pain modulation? A pro-nociceptive shift in central pain modulation may not only carry negative prognostic implications concerning development or progression of chronic pain, it also again requires specific and targeted treatment strategies.

2.1.4 Is Altered Central Nociceptive Processing Still Driven by Peripheral Nociceptive Input?

Normally (some) peripheral nociceptive drive is necessary to maintain (some of the) alterations in central pain processing. There is early evidence that under certain conditions, altered central processing might become autonomous, i.e. no longer dependent on peripheral nociceptive drive. If this is so, this might not only have prognostic connotations, but might also mean that peripheral deafferenting measures will be ineffective, making specific treatment dealing with altered central pain processing mandatory.

The paradigm for our systematic approach to altered pain processing (SATAPP) is summarised below (Figure 5).

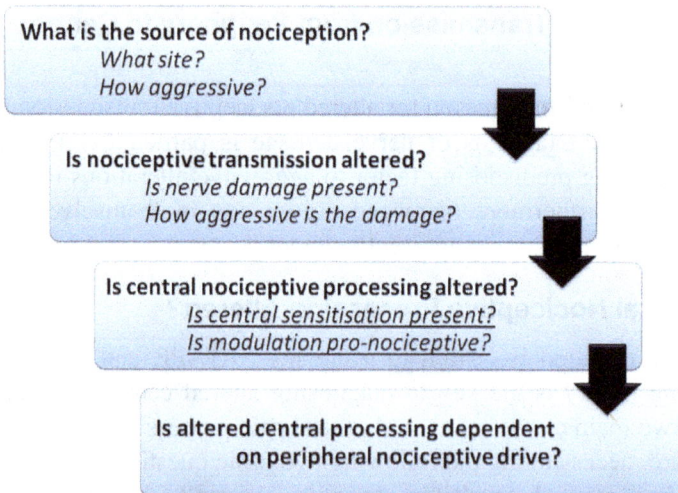

What is the source of nociception?
What site?
How aggressive?

Is nociceptive transmission altered?
Is nerve damage present?
How aggressive is the damage?

Is central nociceptive processing altered?
Is central sensitisation present?
Is modulation pro-nociceptive?

Is altered central processing dependent on peripheral nociceptive drive?

Figure 5   Diagnostic SATAPP paradigm for diagnosing pain disorders

2.2 Diagnostic Needs for SATAPP: QST

As already mentioned, it is now well-recognised that nociception results in altered nervous system sensory processing. Affecting the peripheral and central nervous system, this expresses itself both as alterations in basal pain sensitivity as well as changes in pain modulation. Typically, the initial response is increased pain sensitivity (hyperalgesia), generally rapidly followed by inhibitory modulatory responses[24−26].

In clinical practice it is *impossible* to objectively and reliably diagnose altered pain processing based on symptoms or physical examination alone. There is therefore a real and pressing need for diagnostic technologies permitting the quantification of pain processing in the human clinical context. Quantitative sensory testing (QST) is such a technology. Also termed psychophysical testing, QST is a methodology for systematically quantifying alterations in nervous system sensory function. By formally documenting stimulus-response relationships for pain processing, QST makes visible changes in pain sensitivity and modulation as the basis of a SATAPP in the diagnosis of pain diseases.

QST was initially introduced for neurological sensory diagnosis. In this field, QST is now well-accepted and validated, particularly for the diagnosis of small fibre neuropathy, where it is considered the diagnostic gold standard[51−56]. Later on, QST was introduced into pain medicine, initially to help diagnose neuropathic pain, but now increasingly for the specific purpose of diagnosing the changes in pain processing accompanying nociception and pain. Today QST can be regarded as an established and validated technique, not only specifically for neuropathic pain[53,54,67,68,79], but also for general pain medicine[32,44,45,52,80−85].

2.3 QST Methods for SATAPP

Quantitative sensory testing (QST) has been developed and validated over the last couple of decades as a clinical method in the context of pain disorders for monitoring and diagnosing pain processing, its alterations and its modulation[51−55]. QST can be defined as the determination of stimulus-response relations for nervous system sensory processing under standardised conditions[51,52,55]. Its aim in pain medicine is to formally define the relationships between a stimulus (how strong is the applied stimulus?) and the response (how painful does it feel?), and how these relationships are modulated endogenously and exogenously.

2.3.1 Static QST

Static QST provides information regarding the subject's basal pain sensitivity. This technique is based on the application of defined, usually phasic stimuli to the patient under standardized conditions. The patient is then asked to rate the stimulus regarding its experienced intensity. The use of multiple stimuli with differing intensities makes it possible to construct stimulus-response relationships characterizing the state of the patient's basal pain sensitivity. Increased pain sensitivity, for example, can thus be objectively quantified by the leftward shift it produces (vs. baseline) of the pain stimulus dose-response curve (Figure 6, below)[55].

This procedure is often simplified by determining only one point on the stimulus-response curve, namely a threshold for the transition to pain (the pain threshold) or "intolerable" pain (the pain tolerance threshold). Thresholds are

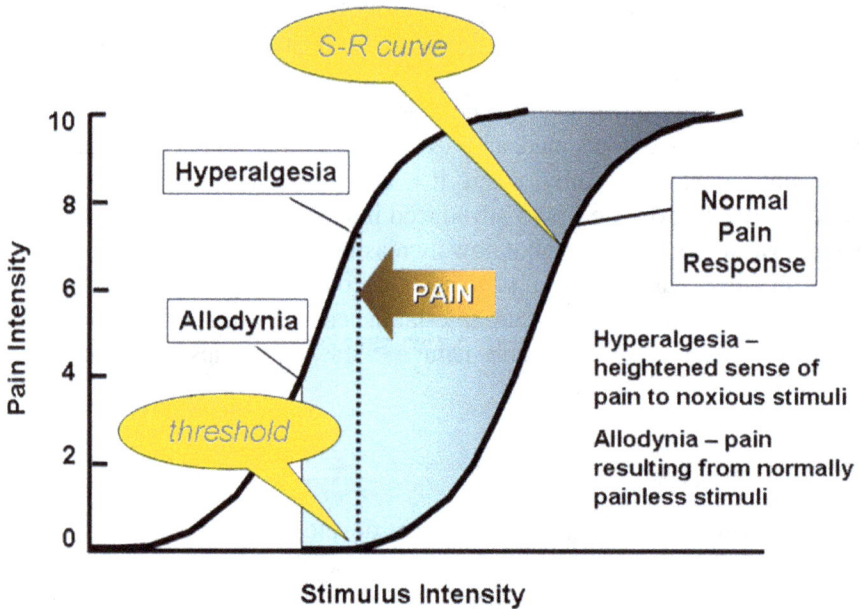

Figure 6 Quantitative sensory testing in pain medicine is based on the construction of a stimulus-response (S-R) curve as illustrated in this figure. The normal S-R curve is shifted to the left by the nociceptive input accompanying pain, causing both hyperalgesia and allodynia. A pain threshold is a defined point on the S-R curve and can thus be used a monoparameter to make visible changes in pain processing such as hyperalgesia or allodynia. Due to the non-linear nature of the S-R relationship, the monoparameter "threshold" will not reliably reflect all aspects of pain processing, e.g. the behaviour of suprathreshold stimulation

a frequently used monoparameter for clinical research into pain processing as it is quick and easy to train patients in their use. The limitations of such a monoparameter, particularly if it does not involve suprathreshold stimulation, must, however, be taken intio account when interpreting it as a measure of pain processing.

Combining different stimulation approaches permits more complete quantification of nociceptive system state under normal and pathophysiological conditions[86,87]. The painful test stimuli can be varied by type, location and tissue stimulated. For "physiological" stimuli (e.g., pressure, temperature, chemical) peripheral nociceptors participate in pain processing. In contrast, electrical stimuli largely bypass nociceptors, reflecting mainly neuronal aspects of nociceptive processing[88,89]. This contrast can be used to provide clues about the state of the peripheral nociceptors and nerves involved in transducing nociceptive inputs.

Stimulation in a variety of anatomical locations (topography) permits conclusions to be drawn about the origin of the altered pain processing within the nervous system. QST measured close to and distant from surgery can, e.g., differentiate between generalised (e.g. supraspinal) and segmental (e.g. spinal) changes in pain processing (I). Combination with different types of stimulation allows further conclusions to be drawn. Examples include secondary or segmental mechanical hyperalgesia indicative of spinal central sensitisation, or thermal hyperalgesia localised to the site of tissue damage with peripheral sensitisation.

Finally, further information can be obtained by stimulating different tissues (e.g. skin, muscle, viscera). Skin – a superficial somatic structure particularly susceptible to sensory modulation – is the most frequently stimulated tissue for QST due to its easy accessibility. Altered pain sensitivity in structures deep to the skin is more difficult to access directly. Such sensitivity may be indirectly studied using cutaneous or muscle projections (e.g. referred areas of viscera)[44,86]. Direct QST of such structures is more invasive and onerous, but can provide additional useful information about altered pain processing in deep structures auch as muscle[44,45] or viscera (e.g. oesophagus[86]).

Combining all of these data will permit the construction of characteristic patterns of altered pain sensitivity associated with various types and stages of pain disorders. At present, QST involving mechanical and electrical stimulation of the skin or mechanical (pressure) stimulation of deeper tissues (muscle, bone) are considered the most reliable and feasible,, and are thus the most frequently used in clinical practice[51,52, 55,56,90,91].

2.3.2 Dynamic QST

QST may be used to test the effect of a conditioning stimulus on the just discussed pain stimulus-response curve. Conditioning may take the form of repeating the (phasic) test stimulus in time or space (Figure 7, below). Such summation informs on mechanisms, e.g. windup, spinal central sensitisation, potentially of relevance to chronic pain and its development[92].

Alternatively, the effects of a variety of (usually tonic and heterotopic) conditioning stimuli on pain processing can be investigated by applying test stimulation before, during and after conditioning stimulation. A typical example is the conditioned pain modulation (CPM) paradigm, also called the diffuse noxious inhibitory controls (DNIC) paradigm[57-62]. CPM is induced via a noxious tonic conditioning stimulus (e.g. cold pressor task) applied remotely from a conditioned test (heterotopic, phasic) pain stimulus, typically resulting in raised pain thresholds and decreased pain perception for the test stimulus[32,60,66,93]. The CPM paradigm (already presented previously in Figure 4) is robust and relatively insensitive to minor details of experimental setup, and makes it possible to visualize the size of descending inhibitory or facilitatory controls – or to gain insight into the pro- vs. antinociceptive balance – in a given patient or patient population[30,31,33,34,59-61,66,75,94-96]. A further

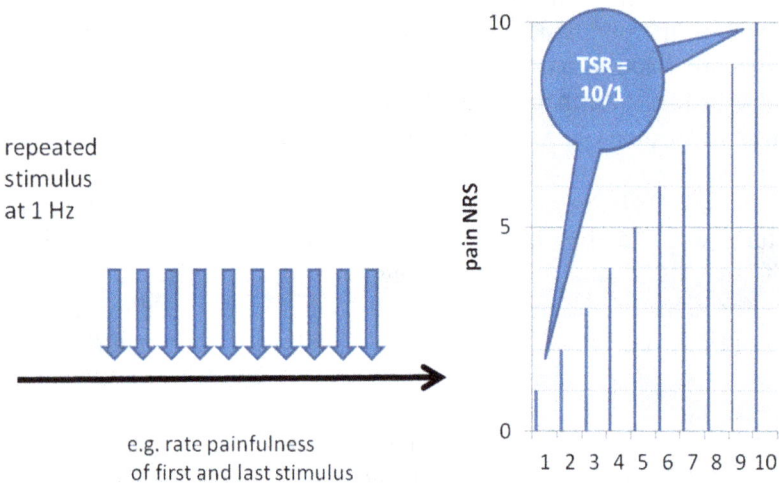

Figure 7 Wind-up paradigm showing effects of temporal summation. Graph on the right shows pain numeric rating score (NRS) for each stimulus; last stimulus of series is more painful than the first, quantified as temporal summation ratio (TSR=NRS for 10th stimulus/1st stimulus)

example is to use high frequency electric cutaneous stimulation as a conditioning stimulus to study the ease of inducing central sensitisation via long-term potentiation[97−101].

2.3.3 QST Interpretation

The results of QST measurements are typically interpreted either in reference to normal values or in reference to the patients' own values before disease or intervention. Normal value databases (e.g. as generated by the German Neuropathic Pain Network[67,68]), are based on QST results obtained in large populations of healthy volunteers of both genders and multiple age ranges, and are scarce due to the considerable resources necessary to generate them. A typical example where a patient can provide his own reference values is in the perioperative context, as many patients are pain-free before surgery and can therefore serve as their own controls[102] (I, II, VI, XIII). Some groups propagate using the side of the body unaffected by pain to provide control values[67,68], but this remains problematic in view of the possibility of spread of altered pain processing to the other side, either due to spread across the spinal cord midline or activation of supraspinal mechanisms.

2.4 Clinical Implementation: The Nijmegen-Aalborg Screening QST (NASQ) Paradigm

As already mentioned above (Figure 5), there are four basic diagnostic questions which form the foundation for a systematic approach to altered pain processing in pain disorders. QST provides results relevant to all four questions.

However question three, i.e. regarding altered central pain processing, is the key question to answer. This is, *firstly*, because the presence of altered central processing has serious prognostic implications for the pain disorder under consideration, and *secondly*, because its presence is often poorly responsive to traditional pain treatments targeting nociceptive input, and requires specific therapeutic measures targeting central pain processing. Moreover, answering question three also provides results relevant to question two (nerve damage can be diagnosed using neurological QST and is typically associated with aggressive changes in central pain processing) and question four (concerning the relationship between altered central processing and peripheral nociceptive input).

A large variety of QST paradigms, both static and dynamic, are available involving different forms of stimulation and different ways of quantifying pain responses. Based on our clinical research experience, we designed a standard screening QST paradigm, the **Nijmegen-Aalborg Screening QST (NASQ)**, suitable for implementation into clinical practice. *My choices* regarding details of the NASQ paradigm were based on 1) what elements of altered pain processing one wants to address and which forms of QST are suitable for this, 2) the scientific evidence that the chosen QST paradigm usefully reflects this aspect of altered pain processing in clinical practice, and 3) practicability and validity for everyday clinical use.

My considerations regarding which forms of altered central pain processing NASQ should first target for clinical use, and the forms of QST suitable for diagnosing these, will be addressed in the following sections of the present chapter. More detailed evidence for the effectiveness of NASQ paradigms in diagnosing altered pain processing in clinical pain practice will be supplied in subsequent chapters dealing with perioperative and chronic pain.

Regarding practicability and validity, our NASQ paradigm characterised below generally lasts about 30 minutes and was well-accepted by patients. Rigid standardisation of the protocols, restriction of measurements to one or two trained personnel, careful initial instruction and training of subjects, and measurement in a quiet secluded room ensured good reproducibility (within 20%) and thus reliability of QST measures.

2.4.1 NASQ and Altered Central Pain Processing: Central Sensitisation

Central sensitisation, both spinal and supraspinal, plays a key role in developing and established chronic pain conditions – a role much more important than peripheral sensitisation. In this context, two types of spread of central sensitisation appears to be particularly linked to development and progression of chronic pain diseases, namely 1) spread of central sensitisation rostrally up the neuraxis, i.e. towards supraspinal or cortical structures, and 2) spread to heterotopic structures or tissues, e.g. from skin to deeper tissues such as muscles. A further reason for detecting central sensitisation is therapeutic: there is accumulating evidence that central sensitisation, once established, responds increasingly poorly to "classic" analgesic measures such as opioid analgesia or peripheral nerve blockade, thus requiring own specific and targeted treatment approaches[103]. Thus the *first* alteration of pain processing which I considered the NASQ paradigm should target is the presence and spread of central sensitisation. A suitable QST paradigm for the detection of central sensitisation and spread should fulfill the following conditions:

1) The ability to detect mechanical hyperalgesia. This is crucial because the secondary hyperalgesia surrounding injured tissue, which is generally considered a definitive manifestation of central sensitisation, is mechanical in nature.
2) The ability to assess spread of central sensitisation. This involves homotopic spread, e.g. to skin distant from the nociceptive source, as well as heterotopic spread, e.g. to muscle, a very important tissue involved in many pain diseases.
3) The ability to quantify pain sensitivity not only at but also above pain threshold. This is important because most clinically relevant pain processing is suprathreshold.

To fulfil these conditions, the NASQ paradigm contains the following elements:

1) Pressure pain thresholds. These mechanical thresholds detect mechanical hyperalgesia of deep tissues such as muscle, thus also permitting assessemtn of heterotopic spread of central sensitisation, and are considered clinically robust and reliable[67,68,104].
2) Electrical detection, pain detection and pain tolerance thresholds. These permit the assessment of skin hyperalgesia, and thus central sensitisation, at and above pain threshold and in comparison with non-nociceptive sensory processing. The ability to stimulate multiple nerve fibre populations and to bypass peripheral nociceptors (and their sensitisation) provides valuable additional insight into more neuronal aspects of pain processing, despite the alleged "unphysiological" nature of the stimulus.
3) Pain thresholds at multiple sites. Multisite measurements allow differentiation between segmental (spinal) vs. generalised (supraspinal) central sensitisation, and the quantification of neuraxial spread of central sensitisation. The minimum of sites is two, one close and one distant from the nociceptive source.

To achieve these ends in clinical practice, I applied simple QST paradigms to determine thresholds via ramping electrical and mechanical stimulation. For *mechanical* stimulation, I used a simple commercially available electronic pressure algometer. Pressure algometry stimulates mainly deeper structures such as muscle, with only a minor contribution from skin processing if used in the classical vertical mode (vs. the pinching mode)[89,105,106]. For *electrical* stimulation we used a simple constant-current device delivering electric tetanic stimuli. Transcutaneous electric stimulation stimulates only superficial cutaneous and subcutaneous structures. It bypasses nociceptors by stimulating cutaneous nerve endings directly, thus providing information on more central aspects of skin pain processing[107,108]. To explore different aspects of nociceptive and non-nociceptive sensory processing, we determined electric sensation (non-nociceptive processing), pain detection and pain tolerance (suprathreshold pain processing) thresholds. Electrical and pressure algometry stimulation were chosen for their ease of use and controllability, as well as for their proven ability to detect both inhibitory and excitatory changes in pain processing[32,46,105,107,109]. Both devices proved reliable and safe in routine clinical use.

The NASQ includes thresholds at multiple sites. For surgical patients, this involved measuring – as a minimum – at one site close to surgical incision and one distant from it. This permits differentiation of generalised (reflecting supraspinal processing) and localised or segmental (reflecting peripheral or spinal processing) changes in pain processing, thus allowing identification of rostral neuraxial spread of altered pain processing in time (I,VI). For the chronic pain patients, we again compared, as a minimum, healthy and affected sites, once more allowing differentiation between segmental and generalised changes in pain processing and their neuraxial spread (I, VI, VIII, IX, XIII, XV). Figure 8 (below) summarises the part of the NASQ paradigm I developed to diagnose spreading central sensitisation, which takes about 20 minutes to perform.

2.4.2 NASQ and Altered Central Pain Processing: Descending Modulation

I had previously mentioned that the central nervous system responds to initial nociceptive input and excitation by generating counteracting inhibition of both spinal and supraspinal origin to depress both noxious spinal inputs and subsequent central sensitisation. In this case, it is generally supraspinal descending modulation which is dominant. There is good evidence, which will be discussed in more detail in subsequent sections, that descending supraspinal modulation, particularly the net balance between pro- and antinociceptive forces, plays a key role in the genesis, progression and prognosis of chronic pain diseases.

In this context a pronociceptive shift of descending pain modulation not only facilitates the entry and ascent of nociceptive signals into the central nervous system, it also favours the rostral spread of central sensitisation up the neuraxis to supraspinal structures, thus ultimately producing the mix of altered nociceptive and non-nociceptive supratentorial processing so

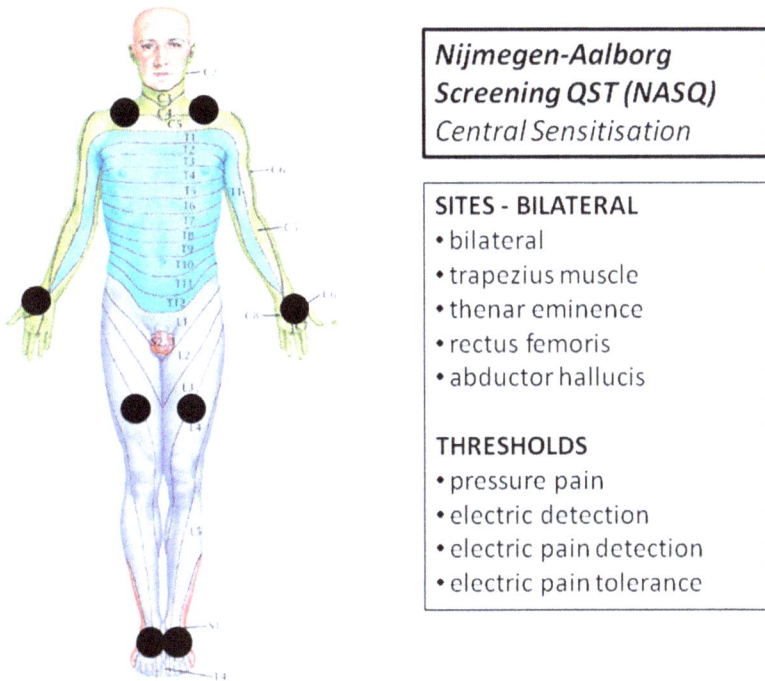

**Nijmegen-Aalborg
Screening QST (NASQ)**
Central Sensitisation

SITES - BILATERAL
• bilateral
• trapezius muscle
• thenar eminence
• rectus femoris
• abductor hallucis

THRESHOLDS
• pressure pain
• electric detection
• electric pain detection
• electric pain tolerance

Figure 8   NASQ part I to detect spreading central sensitisation

characteristic of chronic pain patients. Again there are further, therapeutic reasons for specifically diagnosing altered central pain modulation. Thus there are not only first indications that altered pain modulation responds to different therapeutic manoeuvres than central sensitisation, but also that certain treatments may be less effective in the presence of pronociceptive descending pain modulation.

Thus the *second* alteration of pain processing which I considered the NASQ paradigm should target is the balance between pro- and antinociceptive descending modulation. It should be noted that the presence of descending facilitation is likely to encourage the genesis and spread of central sensitisation. To diagnose descending modulation I used a conditioned pain modulation (CPM) paradigm eliciting a phasic brainstem descending inhibitory control response, diffuse noxious inhibitory controls (DNIC), containing the following elements:

1) An aversive painful, tonic, heterotopic conditioning stimulus. Heterotopy between test and conditioning stimuli ensures maximum supraspinal

processing contribution to the modulatory response; the other conditions ensure that we are dealing with clinically relevant modulation of pain processing.

2) Phasic, heterotopic test stimuli. The reason for heterotopy has already been explained, phasic test stimuli are chosen to minimise the effect which test stimulation has on pain processing. The test stimuli are applied at least before and just after conditioning stimulation to quantify its modulatory effect.

3) Multimodal test stimuli. This is because we cannot necessarily expect descending modulation of different test stimuli to be the same, e.g. for skin vs. muscle.

4) Test stimulation distant and extrasegmental to conditioning site. This ensures that the modulation elicited applies to the entire body, as would be expected for descending controls of supraspinal origin, e.g. DNIC.

I chose the cold pressor task as the tonic painful conditioning stimulus as it is extremely aversive, technically simple to produce and well-validated in the literature[110−113]. Based on the literature, maximum immersion time was limited to 180 seconds, and pain scores pre- and post-immersion documented to assure standardisation of the cold pressor task[112]. The cold pressor task was further selected because it is heterotypic to the test stimuli chosen and also delivers insight into tonic pain sensitivity of the subject via the hand withdrawal latency[112,113]. For test stimulation before and after cold pressor task conditioning we used the same multimodal electric and mechanical test stimuli described above for simple sensitivity testing. Conditioning stimulation was applied to the upper extremity. Test stimulation was carried out on the upper thigh to quantify the distant extrasegmental CPM response, with the response being defined as the percentage change of electrical and pressure pain tolerance threshold after vs. before conditioning (XIII). Figure 9 (below) summarises the part of the NASQ paradigm I developed to diagnose shifts in descending nociceptive modulation, which can be either in the direction of inhibition or in the direction of facilitation. This part of the NASQ paradigm takes about 10 minutes to perform.

2.5 Summary: NASQ Paradigm for SATAPP.QST

Quantitative sensory testing to diagnose alterations in pain sensitivity and modulation is central to achieving rational and effective a systematic approach to altered pain processing in pain disorders. As indicated above, the capacity

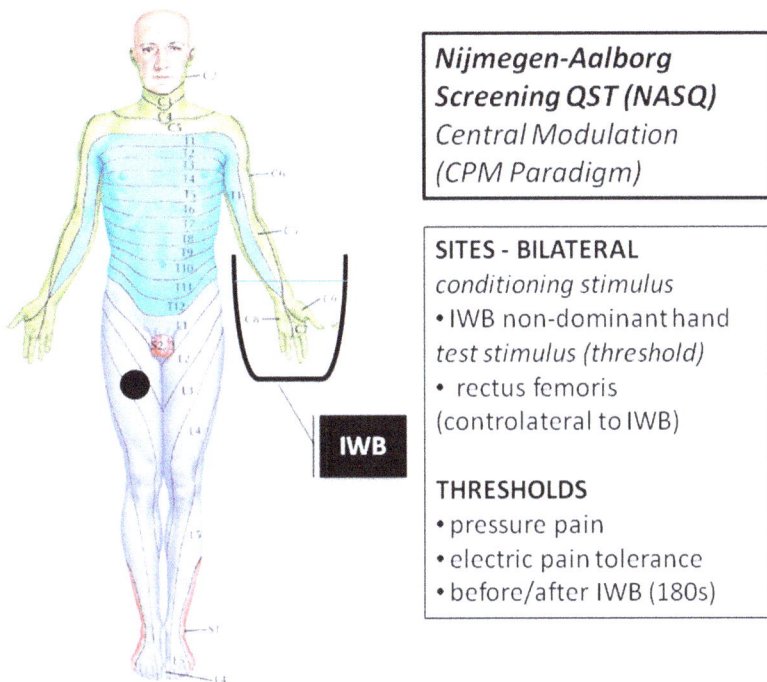

Nijmegen-Aalborg
Screening QST (NASQ)
Central Modulation
(CPM Paradigm)

SITES - BILATERAL
conditioning stimulus
• IWB non-dominant hand
test stimulus (threshold)
• rectus femoris
(controlateral to IWB)

THRESHOLDS
• pressure pain
• electric pain tolerance
• before/after IWB (180s)

IWB

Figure 9 NASQ part II using Conditioned Pain Modulation (CPM) paradigm developed to detect pro-or anti-nociceptive shifts in descending pain modulation. IWB = ice water bucket

of QST to diagnose central sensitisation and altered central pain modulation makes it *key* in answering the questions about altered central pain processing. Thus the diagnosis of central sensitisation and altered pain modulation is central in the design of the Nijmegen-Aalborg Screening QST (NASQ) paradigm. The ability of QST to help diagnose peripheral sensitisation and nerve damage can also be useful in diagnosing peripheral sources of nociceptive input and disorders of nociceptive transmission. In combination with methods to achieve temporary deafferentation of peripheral nociceptive input, QST can help quantify the relationship between the latter and altered central pain processing. In the following chapters covering specific aspects of perioperative and chronic pain, I will provide more detail regarding the role of NASQ in the clinical implementation of a systematic approach to altered pain processing (SATAPP.QST) in pain medicine.

3

SATAPP.QST for Perioperative Practice

3.1 Pain and Surgery

3.1.1 Pain after Surgery: An Ongoing Problem

Post-surgical pain remains a significant and challenging problem. Around 40% of patients experience major acute postoperative pain, about 25% report inadequate pain relief[3]. This situation has not improved over the last 10–15 years despite concerted efforts including the widespread introduction of acute pain services and associated practice guidelines[1–3,5]. For chronic postoperative pain the situation is even less satisfactory, and its significance has only started being appreciated.[4,6−8,114] The literature now becoming available reports incidences of chronic pain of up to 75% for major operations such as amputation or thoracotomy (Table 1)[8]. Even common, relatively minor procedures such as inguinal hernia repair are associated with chronic pain prevalences of up to 30%[6,8,10,11,115−117]. It appears that 10 to 50% of patients complain of chronic pain after surgery, and that this pain is severe, impairs quality of life and is thus significant in 2 to 10% of postoperative patients[8]. Furthermore about a quarter of patients attending a chronic pain outpatient clinic attribute their pain to previous surgery[114]. In summary, pain, particularly chronic pain, is a frequent, clinically relevant and undesirable outcome after surgery that is in urgent need of new, effective medical management approaches. The present section provides a review of the relevant literature regarding the relevance of altered sensory processing to the problem of chronic pain after surgery.

3.1.2 Clinical Risk Factors for Chronic Pain after Surgery and Altered Sensory Processing

What links clinical risk factors associated with higher prevalences of chronic postoperative pain to altered pain processing? Answering this question is

Table 1   Estimated incidence of chronic pain and disability after selected surgical procedures. Modified from reference 8.

	Estimated incidence chronic pain	Estimated incidence severe chronic pain (VAS >5)
Amputation	30–50%	5–10%
Breast surgery	20–30%	5–10%
Thoracotomy	30–40%	10%
Inguinal hernia repair	10%	2–4%
Coronary artery bypass	30–50%	5–10%
Caesarean section	10%	4%

important because, once these links are understood, they may be used to develop and test hypotheses regarding the mechanisms underlying development of, and increased vulnerability to, chronic pain after surgery. In clinical practice, lacking awareness and understanding of underlying alterations in pain processing results impedes the implementation of effective management approaches to surgical pain based on altered pain processing. This in turn helps explain the fact that incidences of acute and chronic postoperative pain continue to be high despite rigorous medical and organizational efforts towards its reduction.

The literature to date has identified a number of risk factors associated with higher prevalences of chronic pain after surgery. These can be grouped into patient-related, surgery-related, psychosocial and socio-environmental aspects. Prominent risk factors in the literature include female gender, younger age, the presence of pre- and postoperative pain, type and extent of surgery, and nerve damage[8,10,11]. All of these factors can be linked to altered pain processing. Thus lower age, consistently associated with higher incidences of chronic postoperative pain, may be associated with a more vigorous neuroplastic response, while gender-dependent differences in pain modulation are now well-described in the literature (XI, XII)[6,8,10,118−120]. Surgery-related risk factors linked to increased incidences of chronic pain after surgery, including more preoperative pain, more pain and higher analgesia consumption in the early postoperative period, more extensive surgery, and nerve damage have increased pain sensitivity in common, in that these factors can all be either expressions of hyperalgesia (more preoperative or postoperative pain, more postoperative analgesia consumption), or a cause thereof (nerve damage, more extensive surgery)[6,8,10,27,118-120]. Other factors associated with higher risk of chronic pain after surgery, e.g. altered genetic status via polymorphisms in relevant genes, or the psychosocial factor of catastrophizing status, are now increasingly discussed in the literature and also linked to altered pain processing[121-138].

3.1.3 Nociception and Central Nervous System Processing in the Surgical Context

It is generally accepted that nociceptive input such as surgery alters pain processing by the nervous system[8,24-27,125,139,140]. This alteration is initially excitatory, usually rapidly followed by inhibitory modulation. In the following sections I briefly summarise the relevance of altered central nervous system processing in the perioperative context to a systematic approach to altered pain processing.

3.1.3.1 Altered nociceptive transmission: nerve damage

I would like to emphasize that the consequences of nociceptive input are more aggressive in the presence of nerve damage than in other contexts such as inflammation. Clinically highly associated with more chronic pain after surgery[8], nociception in the context of nerve damage is also linked to more central sensitization, greater loss of inhibitory controls, and increased descending facilitation[141,142] (Figure 10, below). Such shifts to a pro-nociceptive state not only favour the development of hyperalgesia, they also risk favouring the rostral spread of central sensitisation and the development of changes in central pain processing so characteristic of chronic pain patients.

3.1.3.2 Altered central pain processing: central sensitization

Both peripheral and central pain processing by the nervous system can be sensitised by nociceptive input, a process clinically manifest as hyperalgesia[25-27,139]. Central sensitization is more relevant to clinical pain conditions, and can be the result of 1) enhanced neuronal membrane excitability, 2) increased synaptic efficacy (e.g. via long-term potentiation) and 3) altered modulation in the sense of both disinhibition and facilitation[26,139,]

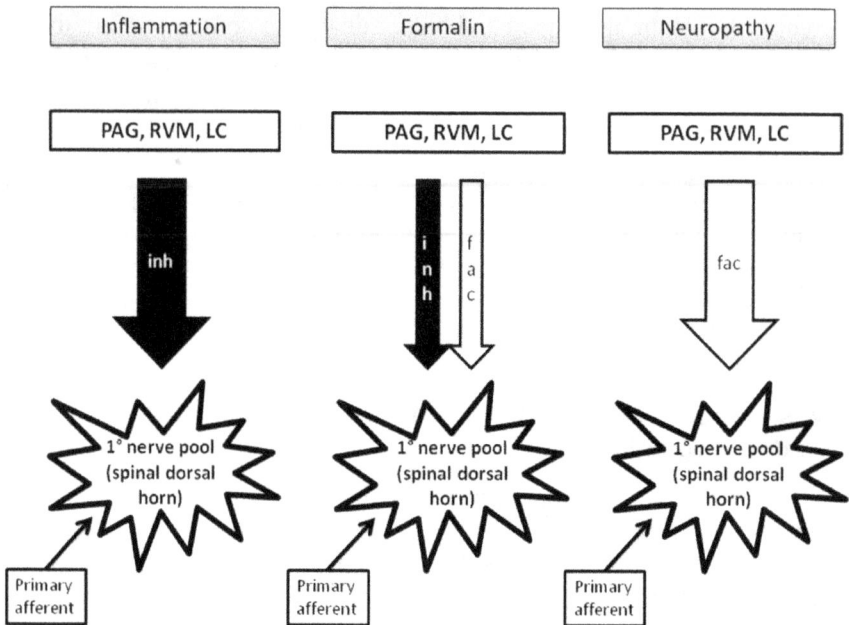

Figure 10   Effects of increasing nerve damage on central processing of afferent nociceptive input. **Inflammation** alone results in strong descending inhibitory modulation (inh) of primary afferent nociceptive input. **Formalin**, which irritates nerves, results in less inhibitory (inh) and more facilitatory (fac) modulation. **Nerve damage (neuropathy)** elicits almost exclusively facilitatory (fac) descending modulation of primary afferent nociceptive input. PAG = peri-aqueductal grey, RVM = rostroventral medulla, LC = locus cereolus. Modified after 141

[143-146]. Persistence and progression of central sensitization as a result of ongoing nociceptive input is considered a central process in the development of chronic pain in the basic animal research literature[24-26,125,139].

With ongoing nociceptive input, central sensitization traverses three increasingly longer-lasting, irreversible and pathological stages, namely activation (transient, activity-dependent), modulation (slower but still reversible functional changes) and modification (chronic structural and architectural alterations)[25]. Activation involves use-dependent augmentation of transduction and transmission (e.g. wind-up) and is a rapidly reversible physiological process[25]. Modulation is a more slowly reversible process with early pathological connotations. It is mainly due to phosphorylation of neuronal receptors and ionophores (e.g. the N-methyl D-aspartate (NMDA) receptor and associated calcium ionophore)[25]. Modification includes altered regulation and cell connectivity together with cell death, and is generally viewed as the basis of chronic, pathological pain. Typically it entails modified gene transcription together with loss of inhibition, both functionally and via death of inhibitory neuron populations[25].

3.1.3.3 Altered central pain processing: central modulation

As previously pointed out, nociceptive input elicits counteracting modulatory responses by the central nervous system. Segmental spinal inhibitory controls, the so-called "spinal gate" of Melzack and Wall[147], represent a first line of defense. Most prominent are the descending inhibitory controls targeting the spinal dorsal horn and thus the first pain pathway synapse, using pathways descending from the brain, particularly from the brainstem[148]. These systems are selective for nociceptive processing, and can be both inhibitory and facilitatory. They are thus decisive for the balance of nociceptive transmission, ultimately determining whether pain processing is in a pro or antinociceptive state[148].

Descending inhibitory control can be broadly divided into three systems:

The *first* is the tonic midline peri-aqueductal grey – rostro-ventral medulla (PAG-RVM) system (of which the locus coeruleus may be considered a part). Its ON- and OFF cells project downwards to the spinal dorsal horn, and facilitate or inhibit nociceptive input, respectively[30,31,141,148,149]. The PAG-RVM system is subject to a variety of supraspinal and cortical modulating inputs[148], and has been demonstrated to control pain sensitivity in a variety of animal models for chronic pain states including arthritis, visceral and neuropathic pain[94,142,148,150].

A *second*, phasic system carries the name "diffuse noxious inhibitory controls" (DNIC). It is based on a spino-bulbo-spinal loop involving the dorsal reticular nucleus of the medulla (DRN)[57,58,60,61,66,151−153]. DNIC can be elicited in animal and humans by applying a local noxious conditioning stimulus which then results in a generalized decrease in pain transmission (the CPM (conditioned pain modulation) paradigm[62,66]), as evidenced by lower evoked pain responses or higher pain thresholds to test stimulation distant from the site of conditioning stimulation[59−61]. The descending inhibition of DNIC affects on spinal dorsal horn wide dynamic range (WDR) neurons of the entire neuraxis, and is considered to not only to be involved in endogenous analgesia but also whole body enteroception, e.g. by improving signal-to-noise ratios for nociceptive input[70].

Supratentorial top-down controls comprise the *third* system. They are believed to be the CNS substrate for the influence of cognitive and affective factors on pain and pain processing, e.g. placebo and nocebo effects[31,141,142,148–150,154–159]. Here higher structures including prefrontal cortex, cingulate cortex, amygdala and hypothalamus have widespread connections with the PAG-RVM system, forming the basis of a variety of central positive and negative feedback loops activated by noxious sensory input[148,154–156,160].

3.1.3.4 Altered central pain processing: dependence on peripheral nociceptive input

There are indications that after aggressive and/or long-lasting ongoing nociceptive input the ensuing alterations to central pain processing become progressively less dependent on the initiating afferent nociceptive input[161,162]. If this is so, then autonomous central processing independent of peripheral nociceptive input could represent the end stage of the process of chronic pain development. This topic is dealt with in more detail in the next chapter.

3.2 Synopsis of Own Contributions

Eight of my articles included in this review deal with the perioperative situation. In these articles I define the problem of perioperative pain, document the time course of perioperative alterations in pain processing, and investigate the perioperative factors influencing postoperative pain outcomes.

3.2.1 Defining the Problem

In a large survey of perioperative and emergency room analgesia in Switzerland (IV) I attempted to define the problems as perceived by the doctors practicing in this area. Encouragingly, the majority of the doctors questioned were convinced of the key contribution which effective perioperative pain management makes to better long-term pain outcomes after surgery. However, I was able to identify serious problems and concerns concentrated in two main areas, namely education and organisation. Thus less than half the respondents said they had undergone—or were undergoing – structured or accredited pain education, and less than a third participated in regular educational meetings with the goal of providing ongoing training and providing feedback and troubleshooting for pain management problems in everyday perioperative practice. Regarding organisation, less than a third of respondents regularly determined pain scores in the perioperative context, only some 15% performed regular analysis of pain outcomes in the context of a quality assurance programme, and barely 10% had standard treatment plans (algorithms) in place upon which to base postoperative analgesic management. None of the respondents formally assessed sensory processing in the perioperative context.

We further studied the influence of nerve damage on chronic pain incidence after breast cancer surgery (XI). It is well-known that axillary lymph node dissection is associated with surgical damage to large nerves traversing the axilla. In a large retrospective survey of patients having undergone breast cancer surgery we documented that concomitant axillary lymph node dissection doubled the prevalence of chronic pain from 23% to 51%. Moreover, axillary lymph node dissection also interacted with both postoperative chemo- and radiotherapy to further increase the risk of chronic pain. These results strongly support a major role of nerve damage in the genesis of chronic pain after surgical interventions.

Thoracic surgery is associated with a high incidence of chronic pain[8]. This high incidence is again considered to be the result of nerve damage, incurred as a result of rib retraction during thoracotomy. In a large retrospective study of thoracic surgery, I was able to confirm the high prevalence of chronic pain (XII). However comparison of chronic pain prevalences for open thoracotomy (40%) and for thoracoscopic procedures (47%) suggests that nerve damage may not be the only factor explaining high incidences of persisting pain after surgery, as thoracoscopy does not involve rib retraction, significantly reducing the likelihood of nerve damage. This finding is supported by the results from the use in my study of a validated screening questionnaire for neuropathic pain in these patients, which showed that only 23% of these patients had definite signs of neuropathic pain, while 47% showed no signs of neuropathic pain. Thus it is likely that other sources of poorly modulated nociceptive input, e.g. visceral nociception accompanying thoracic surgery, also play a significant role in increasing risk of persisting or chronic pain after surgery.

3.2.2 Time Course of Altered Sensory Processing after Surgery

Few other studies have systematically investigated the time course or topography of altered pain processing after surgery. My research has produced the only published documentation to date of the long-term time course of altered postoperative pain processing, involving multiple QST measurements from one hour up to six months after surgery. This is the first time long-term monitoring of altered pain processing using a multimodal QST paradigm such as NASQ has been shown to be feasible in the clinical context.

Furthermore, my studies are the only ones to have assessed heterotopic spread of altered central processing by measuring both electrical thresholds, reflecting skin sensitivity (without nociceptor contribution) and mechanical pressure pain thresholds, reflecting deep tissue (e.g. muscle) sensitivity (I, II, VI, XIII). My studies are further unique in having measured thresholds at multiple sites to differentiate peri-incisional (i.e. secondary) hyperalgesia from spreading changes in pain processing expressed as generalised hyperalgesia. In particular, our studies appear to be the only ones to systematically investigate the phenomenon of generalised hyperalgesia. This is important as peri-incisional changes will reflect mainly altered spinal processing, while generalised changes will tend to reflect supraspinal mechanisms. The distinction is key because in comparison to spinal sensitisation, supraspinal spread of central sensitisation, *firstly*, has more pathological connotations regarding chronic pain development, *secondly*, is more difficult to reverse, and *thirdly*, has more extensive effects on other aspects of CNS processing[24–27,30,31,33,35,43,142,149,150,163,164].

My studies show that during the first 24 postoperative hours, inhibitory changes as revealed by electric skin pain thresholds predominate. The fact that inhibition affected all sensory modalities, including non-nociceptive ones, tends to speak against morphine effects, as opioids mainly affect tonic pain stimuli corresponding to pain tolerance thresholds and C-fibre transmission, leaving A-beta fibre mediated non-nociceptive sensory transmission unchanged[165,166]. Thus we suggest this acute, inhibition is likely due to tonic descending inhibitory controls, e.g. from the PAG-RVM system[148,] acting on spinal wide dynamic range neurons[167]. This view is supported by the generalised and acute nature of the inhibition and its effects on both nociceptive and non-nociceptive sensory modalities[152,167,168]. The level adaptation theory suggests that pain thresholds change due to reference point resetting, but is disqualified by the parallel changes in non-nociceptive processing seen in our studies[169].

From day one to the end of the first postoperative week, excitatory changes can become visible, with peri-incisional and spreading/generalised hyperalgesia increasing considerably from postoperative day 1 to 5 (I, II, VI, XIII). This *increase* in hyperalgesia occurs parallel to a *reduction* of pain scores and analgesia consumption, again underlining the general lack of correlation between clinical pain measures and QST measures found in our – and others' – research. The results suggest that spread of central sensitisation up the neuraxis to supraspinal structures can occur quite early – i.e. the first few postoperative days – and that it is not well reflected in clinical pain measures. Of note is that – under some circumstances – the presence of substantial descending inhibitory controls during the first 24 hours is not enough to prevent this subsequent spread from occurring. Certainly nerve damage seems to play an important role in this context, as my studies show spreading/generalised hyperalgesia on postoperative day five in back surgery patients (who often show nerve damage), but not in hysterectomy patients (who generally do not have nerve damage).

Other studies have described peri-incisional secondary mechanical hyperalgesia from 24 hours up to 7 days after surgery[37−42], congruent with our results using electrical stimulation (I, VI, XIII). Only two of the quoted studies determined pressure pain thresholds[37,39], the others quantified hyperalgesia by mapping the area of punctuate hyperalgesia (i.e. secondary hyperalgesia) around surgical incision[38,40−42]. Using mapping after abdominal surgery, one group found peri-incisional hyperalgesia areas to increase from postoperative day 1 to 3[40−42]. These results are compatible with our findings, particularly in view of the strong correlation we found between peri-incisional and generalised hyperalgesia (I, VI, XIII).

My research is unique in having extended the period of QST monitoring of altered sensory processing to six months after surgery (XIII). We have shown that, for major abdominal surgery, patients *without* chronic pain at six months do not in general show significant postoperative hyperalgesia of the skin or muscle during their six month postoperative course. In contrast, patients *with* chronic pain six months postoperatively demonstrate persistence of both skin and muscle hyperalgesia – from one day up to six months postoperatively. Both pain experience (i.e. VAS for pain) and pain processing (hyperalgesia spread) postoperatively were affected by the inhibitory effectiveness of preoperative pain modulation. Thus greater preoperative inhibition of skin nociceptive inputs reduced postoperative persistent pain VAS, while greater preoperative inhibition of muscle/deep tissue nociceptive inputs reduced postoperative spreading deep tissue hyperalgesia.

Remarkably, postoperative hyperalgesia from day one to three months postoperatively in the group with chronic pain was not accompanied by higher pain VAS; increased VAS were only seen at six months, again demonstrating the only weak link between subjective measures of pain experience and measures of altered pain processing. These results suggest that the development of chronic pain after surgery is linked to the persistence and rostral spread of neuraxial central sensitisation, and that this process can start early, i.e. days after surgery. Furthermore, it would appear that the changes in supratentorial pain processing which underlie the altered subjective pain experience of

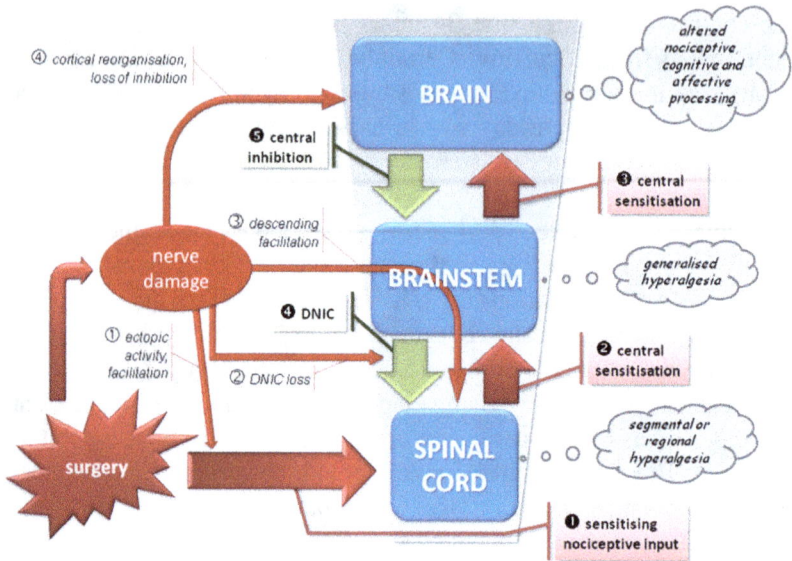

Figure 11   This schematic illustrates the concept of progressive neuraxial spread of central sensitisation (progression numbered by black-filled circles) following ongoing nociceptive inputs due to the tissue and nerve damage (consequences numbered via unfilled circles) of surgery. Note that each stage of rostral spread of central sensitisation is subject to descending modulation

chronic pain takes some time, i.e. months after surgery, to develop. This concept is summarised in Figure 11, below.

3.2.3 Preoperative Factors and Postoperative Pain Outcomes

A number of studies have found preoperative pain ratings evoked by suprathreshold tonic thermal stimuli to predict early postoperative pain scores – but without studying effects on postoperative hyperalgesia[110,137,170,171]. My studies are the only ones to systematically investigate the preoperative prediction of early postoperative hyperalgesia using QST. Thus I found preoperative pain tolerance thresholds in an area distant from back surgery to be a strong factor predicting generalised hyperalgesia from 24 hours to 5 days postoperatively. Here low preoperative pain tolerance thresholds (i.e. high sensitivity to phasic pain stimulation) were found to correlate with less generalised hyperalgesia postoperatively. In the one study where we examined this phenomenon in more detail (VI), we further found this relationship to be disrupted by pre-emptive opioid supplementation, suggesting that such supplementation prevented the state change driving the relationship between preoperative pain thresholds and subsequent generalised hyperalgesia. This result is in line with the previously discussed concept of preemptive analgesia by opioids and the prevention of the central nervous system state change of central sensitisation[25,71,172–175].

The relationship between low preoperative pain tolerance thresholds and decreased early postoperative hyperalgesia may appear counterintuitive at first. Because we did not measure CPM/DNIC in this early study, we can only speculate that perhaps a lower (phasic) pain threshold in a person with a healthy pain processing system leaves more room for dynamic inhibitory processes than if the threshold is higher. This is supported by recent studies indicating a ceiling effect for the DNIC response elicited when using the CPM paradigm[60]. If true, this would associate higher thresholds with decreased ability to produce DNIC or other inhibitory modulation. However, the relationship between CPM responses and basal pain thresholds has not been reported to date for healthy persons. Alternatively, a higher threshold might simply be associated with more tonic inhibition to lose. Clearly more specific research targeting this area is necessary. Our studies do suggest (particularly study VI), however, that it should now be possible to estimate a cut-off point for preoperative pain tolerance thresholds above which the risk of developing generalised early postoperative hyperalgesia is significantly present, and that this cut-off point will vary with the surgical procedure and type of analgesic supplementation of anaesthesia.

In another study (study V), I demonstrated that the presence of low back pain is associated with more generalised hyperalgesia, in keeping with the results from other studies[45,78,176,177]. In the context of back pain patients undergoing back surgery (I, VI), I also found that the presence and degree of preoperative low back pain influenced the incidence – but not the degree – of generalised hyperalgesia in the first postoperative week[178]. The effect of preoperative pain was large, doubling the incidence of significant generalised hyperalgesia in the first postoperative week. Taking these two results together, we suggest that it is the preoperative hyperalgesia accompanying preoperative back pain which contributes to the increased vulnerability of these patients to generalised hyperalgesia in the early postoperative period after back surgery. These considerations would also help explain the poor outcomes of back surgery for chronic low back pain[15,16,19,20,22,23,179,180].

In the human pain research literature, impaired inhibitory pain modulation ability (e.g. CPM/DNIC response) has been connected to risk or presence of chronic pain[32–34,46,181,182]. Furthermore, impaired inhibitory controls are also linked to the presence of hyperalgesia, a process in which descending facilitation also plays an important role[31−33,43,183]. It would thus appear logical to postulate that weaker preoperative inhibitory modulatory responses (e.g. measured via CPM/DNIC paradigm) might increase the risk of developing generalised hyperalgesia and thus persistent and chronic pain after an acute nociceptive episode such as surgery. Both of these suggestions are supported by our study on abdominal surgery and chronic pain, which not only links chronic pain to poorer skin CPM responses, but also links heterotopic spread of hyperalgesia to poorer deep tissue CPM responses (XIII). Further support is provided by another study where poor preoperative skin CPM responses were associated with more chronic pain after thoracotomy[95].

In summary, our studies have identified three factors, i.e. 1) high basal pain tolerance thresholds, 2) generalised hyperalgesia due to chronic pain disorders as well as 3) poor inhibitory descending pain modulation as significant preoperative predictors of postoperative risk of spreading hyperalgesia and its subsequent persistence. Spreading and persisting hyperalgesia is in turn linked to poor longer-term pain outcomes.

3.2.4 Intra- and Early Postoperative Factors and Postoperative Pain Outcomes

In my studies, *effective antinociception* started before surgery reduced postoperative spreading hyperalgesia. Thus opioid analgesic supplementation of anaesthesia started preoperatively improved inhibitory responses for the first 24 postoperative hours after back surgery for all sensory modalities. Furthermore, such pre-emptive analgesia was subsequently able to prevent significant postoperative hyperalgesia from developing (i.e. reductions in pain tolerance thresholds in the first postoperative week (I, II, VI)). However, opioids started postoperatively and continued for 24 hours were not able to subsequently prevent such spreading hyperalgesia (I, VI). Taken together, these findings suggest that opioids given before nociceptive surgical input starts are able to sufficiently inhibit nociception (perhaps together with acute endogenous inhibitory responses) to prevent subsequent spinal central sensitisation and its progression up the neuraxis to become visible as spreading hyperalgesia. Conversely, opioids started after surgery are not sufficiently potent with regard to depressing established central sensitisation[103] to prevent its subsequent neuraxial spread and expression as spreading or generalised hyperalgesia. These results are in keeping with the neurophysiological evidence from animal experiments for the phenomenon of pre-emptive analgesia[25,72,175,184,] and represent the first true clinical proof of its reality. To our knowledge, only one other study has formally demonstrated the effectiveness of pre-emptive parenteral opioids using QST to date[185].

Another group has studied long-term effects (up to 1 year postoperatively) regarding pain outcomes of *antihyperalgesic treatment* using intravenous ketamine infusion combined with continuous epidural analgesia in abdominal surgery patients. This study showed decreased areas of peri-incisional hyperalgesia up to three days postoperatively and less chronic pain up to six months after surgery using a perioperative intravenous infusion of ketamine[40]. This study did not, however, investigate prediction of postoperative hyperalgesia or pain based on preoperative QST findings (e.g. via pain thresholds or CPM/DNIC paradigm). These results are in agreement with other studies of postoperative pain processing after perioperative use of ketamine[37,38,40,41,186,187,] and are congruent with the generally beneficial effects of ketamine on postoperative pain outcomes[186,188−192]. The group found similar results for intrathecal clonidine, suggesting that both ketamine and clonidine may be effective in reducing acute and chronic rostral neuraxial spread of central sensitisation in the context of chronic pain development.

Further re-analysis of my studies[178] (I, II, VI) would suggest that the incidences of significant spreading hyperalgesia in the first postoperative week (i.e. pain threshold reduction greater than 25% vs. preoperatively) were generally greater for back surgery than hysterectomy (24 hours postoperatively: 24% vs. 3%; 5 days postoperatively: 67% vs. 40%; respectively). However, the hysterectomy patients had no pain preoperatively, and on comparing back patients without preoperative pain with hysterectomy patients, similar incidences of generalised hyperalgesia are found (24 hours: 8% vs. 3%; 5 days: 44% vs. 40%; respectively). We have found no other studies formally investigating the effect of different types of surgery on postoperative pain processing to date.

In summary, my studies in conjunction with others suggest that effective antinociception, antihyperalgesia and type of surgery influence postoperative spread and persistence of hyperalgesia, and thus contribute to better long-term postoperative pain outcomes.

3.2.5 Late Postoperative Factors and Postoperative Pain Outcomes

Our research is the first to link the development of chronic pain after surgery to the persistence and spread of hyperalgesia postoperatively. My results show that patients developing chronic pain six months after surgery show persistent and spreading hyperalgesia at one, three and six months after surgery, particularly of skin, but also of deep tissues such as muscle. Based on these data, which are compatible with the neuraxial persistence and spread of central sensitisation, we would suggest that the presence of heterotopic spreading hyperalgesia beyond the first week or so after surgery indicates an increased risk for the later development of chronic pain. Our data further suggest that alterations in purely nociceptive processing, which tend to involve more caudal neuraxial central sensitisation, predate the changes in pain experience typical of chronic pain, with its characteristic additional alterations in non-nociceptive processing (e.g. cognitive, affective) and effects on more rostral aspects of nociceptive processing. Clearly, further research will be necessary, *firstly* to confirm the innovative hypotheses generated by our research, and *secondly*, to validate resulting sensitive biomarkers documenting the risk of developing chronic pain.

3.3 Synthesis of Current Knowledge: Altered Pain Processing Before and After Surgery

The following paragraphs summarise and systematize what is now known – also as based on the contributions of my perioperative research – about perioperative alterations in pain processing as the basis for realising SATAPP.QST in the perioperative period.

3.3.1 Preoperative Period

Hyperalgesia is increasingly documented in patients preoperatively. Surgery for chronic low back pain is linked to poor chronic pain outcomes[17,20,22,179,180,193−196]. In the context of back surgery for intervertebral disc prolapse, patients with low back pain preoperatively were significantly hyperalgesic just before surgery compared to those without pain preoperatively (V). Those patients with preoperative pain also had a significantly higher incidence of generalized hyperalgesia at the end of the first postoperative week (Figure 12, below)[178].

Similarly, patients awaiting hip replacement surgery for chronic pain due to osteoarthritis, demonstrate not only generalized hyperalgesia, but also impaired inhibitory controls during CPM paradigm[32]. Interestingly, hyperalgesia and poor inhibitory controls reverted to normal in the pain-free state six

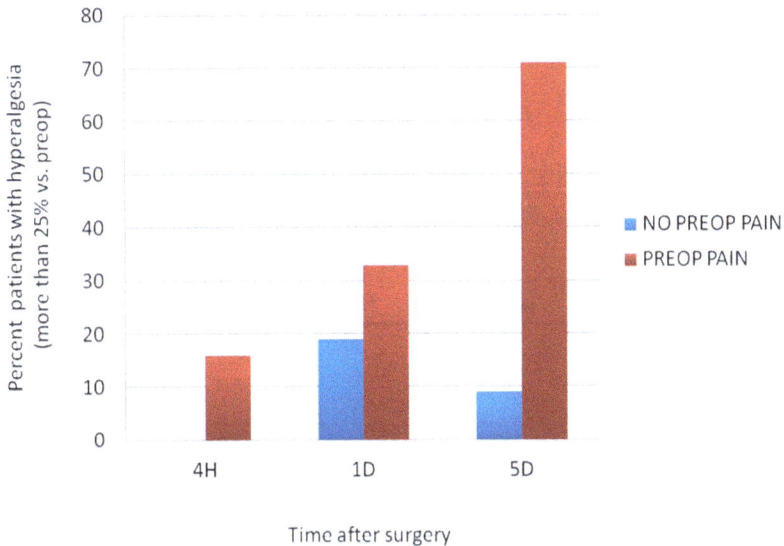

Figure 12   Effects of presence or absence of preoperative pain on incidence (in percent) of postoperative hyperalgesia greater than 25% (vertical axis) in back surgery patients. Horizontal axis gives hours (H) or days (D) postoperatively. Modified after reference[178]

months after hip replacement surgery[32]. This suggests that in these patients, central alterations in pain processing were still beinig driven by peripheral nociceptive input, and thus disappeared with effective treatment of the source of pain.

From the discussion above, poor inhibitory modulation of pain processing preoperatively might be expected to be linked to greater risk of persisting or chronic pain after surgery. Indeed, for thoracic surgery, a key study for the first time directly linked poor preoperative inhibitory pain modulation (CPM paradigm) and higher incidences of chronic pain 30 weeks postoperatively[95]. For major abdominal surgery, my group has confirmed this result, linking the presence of chronic pain six months after surgery to poorer preoperative inhibitory pain modulation of the skin (CPM paradigm using electric skin pain thresholds). In addition, I was able to demonstrate that the persistence of heterotopically spreading hyperalgesia (mechanical muscle pain thresholds in the leg) up to three months postoperatively (Figure 13, below) as a sign of rostral neuraxial spread and persistence of central sensitisation was also linked to poorer preoperative inhibitory pain modulation, this time of the muscle (CPM paradigm using mechanical muscle pain thresholds) (XIII).

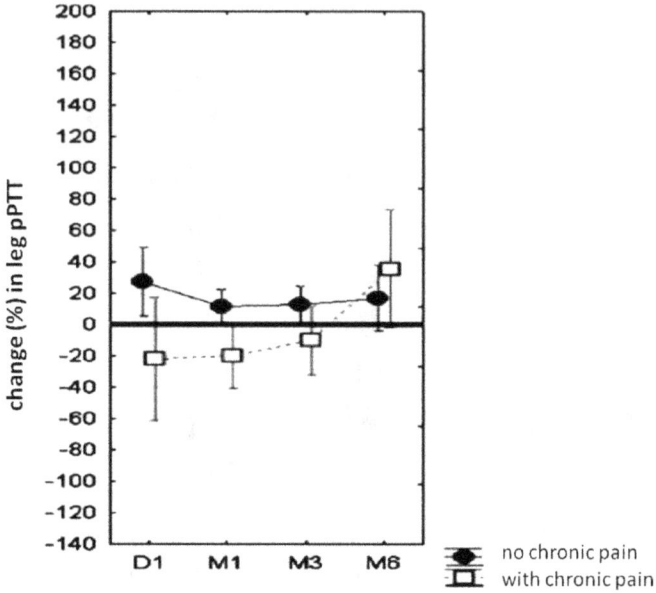

Figure 13   Patients with chronic pain six months after major abdominal surgery (with CP) show persisting spreading heterotopic hyperalgesia (measured in leg muscle using pressure pain tolerance thresholds, pPTT) for the first three months postoperatively, while patients without chronic pain (no CP) do not. Degree of heterotopic hyperalgesia in the leg was inversely correlated with preoperative inhibitory modulation of leg pressure pain thresholds (CPM paradigm). Values are means and 95% confidence intervals. Modified after dissertation reference XIII

In summary, we now possess evidence that generalized hyperalgesia and poor inhibitory modulation are present preoperatively in some patient groups at high risk for postoperative chronic pain development. These changes in pain processing resemble those present in chronic pain patients. Poor preoperative inhibitory modulation has been directly linked not only to increased incidences of chronic pain after surgery, but also to persistent spreading hyperalgesia indicative of supraspinal central sensitisation after surgery. These findings further emphasize the importance of preoperative QST screening via NASQ to achieve SATAPP.QST in the surgical context and thus improve long-term outcomes after surgery.

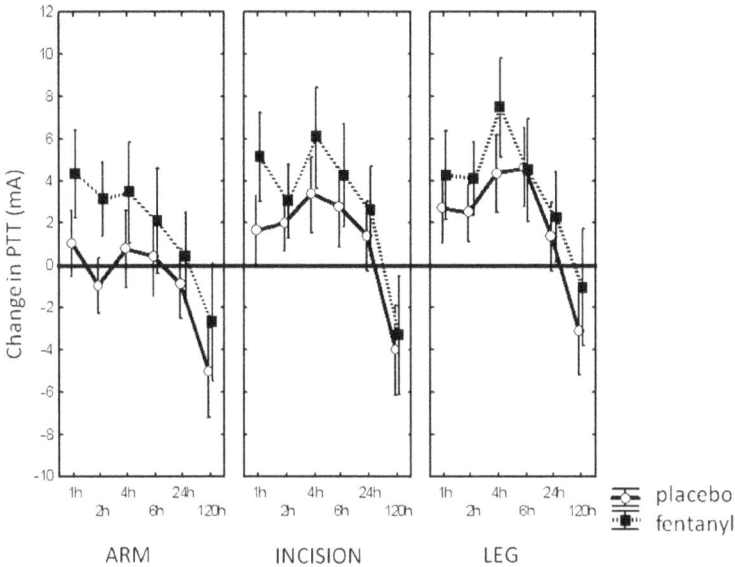

Figure 14 Patients after back surgery show a predominantly hypoalgesic response, greater in the presence of analgesic opioid (fentanyl) supplementation, for the first 24 hours postoperatively. Five days postoperatively, significant segmental and spreading hyperalgesia appears, predominantly in the placebo group. Vertical axis shows change in electric pain tolerance thresholds vs. preoperatively (in mA). The upper horizontal axis shows time postoperatively in hours; the lower horizontal axis shows site of threshold measurement (arm, peri-incisionally, leg). Values are means and 95% confidence intervals. Modified after dissertation reference I

3.3.2 Early Postoperative Period: First Week

Our studies demonstrate that the first 24 hours after surgery are dominated by generalized skin hypoalgesia, probably reflecting descending inhibitory modulation, and greater with better intraoperative analgesia (Figure 14, below) (I, II, VI). Hypoalgesia decreases subsequently, becoming overt generalized hyperalgesia by postoperative day 5 in back surgery – but not abdominal surgery – patients (I, II, VI). The generalized hyperalgesia in back surgery patients at the end of the first week is reduced by pre-emptive opioids, but not by NSAIDs such as ketorolac (I, VI). Such early hyperalgesia is also increased in patients reporting pain preoperatively, as mentioned earlier[178]. This hyperalgesia is likely a reflection of the now well-documented, frequent neuropathic elements in back pain[194−196] and their resulting undesirable effects on passive and active pain processing, typically relatively resistant to opioid therapy[53,140,197−199].

Surgical incision is surrounded by hyperalgesic skin in the early postoperative period (from day 1 of the first postoperative week) as a reflection of spinal central sensitisation[40]. This area increases in size at least up to the third day postoperatively and is decreased by effective perioperative antinociception such as epidural analgesia, or by antihyperalgesic drugs such as ketamine or clonidine[40–42]. Increased *areas* of such peri-incisional (or secondary) hyperalgesia have now been demonstrated to be associated with higher rates of chronic pain up to one year after abdominal surgery[40–42].

Our group has demonstrated that the *degree* of early peri-incisional (secondary) hyperalgesia after surgery (i.e. thresholds) is also decreased by a variety of analgesic drugs as supplements to intraoperative anaesthesia (I, VI). In these studies we were additionally able to demonstrate the presence of spreading/generalised hyperalgesia. This finding is compatible with supraspinal central sensitisation already being present in the early postoperative period, and was also affected by intraoperative analgesic supplementation.

Furthermore, we have also for the first time linked greater *degrees* of hyperalgesia in the early postoperative period to the presence of chronic pain six months after abdominal surgery (XIII). Of note is the fact that this link applies not only to secondary skin hyperalgesia, but equally to spreading or generalised skin hyperalgesia. Moreover, greater degrees of spreading or generalised hyperalgesia were also seen heterotopically, namely in mechanical muscle pain thresholds. This suggests that supraspinal spread of central sensitisation can occur early in a subgroup of patients susceptible to chronic pain after surgery.

Of note is the fact that in all of the studies cited, there is only a weak correlation between postoperative changes in pain processing, as detected by QST, and postoperative clinical measures of pain experience, such as pain VAS or analgesia consumption. Thus the detection of hyperalgesia in the clinical context requires the performance of formal QST and cannot reliably be inferred from clinical measures of the pain experience[40–42] (I, II, VI, XIII).

In summary, there is accumulating data about hyperalgesia – both secondary and generalized – in the first week after surgery as a reflection of spinal and supraspinal central sensitisation. Extent and degree of hyperalgesia are favourably influenced by antinociceptive and antihyperalgesic interventions. In surgical patient groups vulnerable to poor long-term pain outcomes, spread of central sensitisation to supraspinal centres can occur early. My group has presented first evidence that links greater extent and degree of early postoperative hyperalgesia with more chronic pain later on. Thus QST monitoring of spread and persistence of hyperalgesia using NASQ in the early postoperative period is fundamental to achieving better pain outcomes after surgery in the context of perioperative SATAPP.

3.3.3 Late Postoperative Period: Months to Year

Few studies documenting longer-term altered pain processing after surgery have been published to date. Some studies are available linking hyperalgesia at a given time point after surgery with the presence of chronic pain, including mastectomy, hip replacement, maxillofacial or inguinal hernia surgery[118,200,201]. Sensory findings compatible with nerve damage are often also demonstrated in these studies. My group has recently documented the time course of pain and altered pain processing for six months after abdominal surgery (XII) (Figure 15, below). Postoperative pain VAS was negatively correlated with preoperative pain modulation (CPM/DNIC) of the skin, particularly at six months. Patients with chronic pain six months postoperatively showed consistently more peri-incisional and spreading/generalized skin hyperalgesia over the six-month postoperative period. The chronic pain group also displayed more distant deep tissue hyperalgesia. This hyperalgesia was negatively correlated with preoperative inhibitory deep tissue pain modulation. Of note was that differences in postoperative pain VAS between groups reporting pain or no pain six months after surgery only became apparent and significant from three months postoperatively.

The data presently available regarding pain processing in the late postoperative period suggests that patients suffering persistent, chronic pain after surgery exhibit spinal and supraspinal central sensitisation, manifest as peri-incisional and generalized hyperalgesia. This finding is similar to the changes in sensory processing found in patients suffering chronic pain of non-surgical origin.

In summary, we now possess first evidence that chronic pain development after surgery is associated with heterotopic (affecting both skin and deep tissue) persistence and spread of hyperalgesia. Both increased pain experience and hyperalgesia spread appear to be favoured by poor inhibitory pain modulation preoperatively. There is again a lack of correlation between objective measures of altered pain processing and subjective reported pain experience. All of these factors indicate the importance of ongoing QST monitoring for hyperalgesia and pro-nociceptive modulation using NASQ to achieve effective SATAPP.QST and improve pain outcomes in the late postoperative period.

3.4 Summary: Clinical Perioperative Application of SATAPP.QST

In summary, my perioperative pain research distinguishes itself by being the first to investigate the dynamic spreading and heterotopic nature of the sensory phenomena involved over a long postoperative follow-up period, regarding not only central sensitisation, but also its inhibitory modulation. My research using NASQ has provided strong initial evidence to support the key role of persistence and spread of hyperalgesia during the development of chronic pain after surgery, and for the increased risk caused in this context by poor preoperative inhibitory modulation of pain processing as measured by CPM/DNIC paradigm. Furthermore, my research has confirmed the negative role of nerve damage and preoperative central sensitisation (expressed as pain and hyperalgesia) in this context.

Some important conclusions regarding the relevance of NASQ for achieving clinical implementation of SATAPP.QST can be drawn as a result:

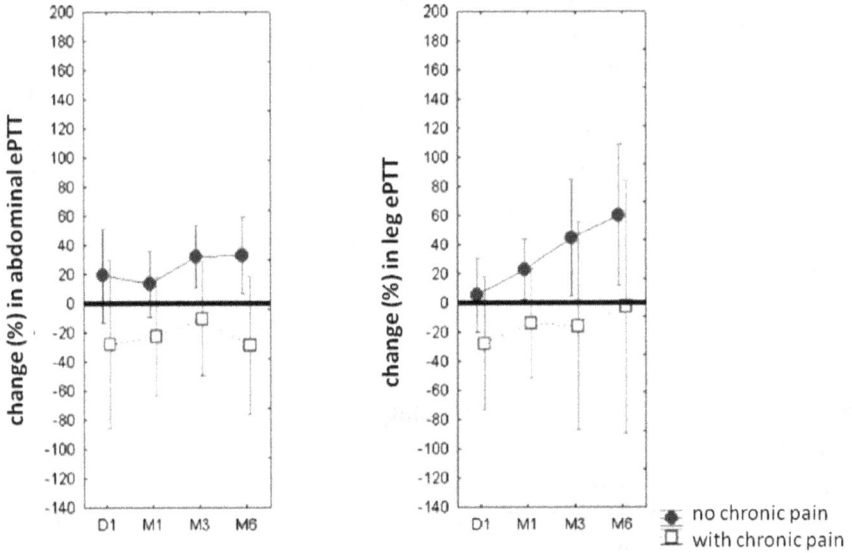

Figure 15 Patients with chronic pain six months after major abdominal surgery (with CP) show persisting secondary and spreading skin hyperalgesia (measured in abdominal and leg skin using electric pain tolerance thresholds, ePTT) for the first six months postoperatively, while patients without chronic pain (no CP) do not. Values are means and 95% confidence intervals. Modified after dissertation reference XIII

Firstly, pre-operative determination of effectiveness of inhibitory pain modulation via CPM/DNIC paradigm may be a predictive biomarker for risk of chronic pain development.

Secondly, monitoring of persistence and spread of hyperalgesia after surgery may be a useful biomarker of ongoing vulnerability to chronic pain development. The risk for hyperalgesia appears to increase with pre/intratraoperative nerve damage and central sensitisation.

Thirdly, it appears logical to posit that risk of developing chronic pain after surgery is decreased by therapeutic measures to diminish persistence and spread of hyperalgesia. This may be achieved by reducing nociceptive input and/or by targeting hyperalgesia, either directly by antihyperalgesic treatments or indirectly by improving inhibitory controls.

Finally, implementation of these conclusions in everyday clinical practice is impossible without objectively diagnosing altered pain sensitivity (hyperalgesia) and pain modulation (CPM paradigm) – and this is impossible without implementing QST diagnostics into clinical practice. e.g. via NASQ. My research demonstrates importance and value of perioperative QST monitoring in clinical pain practice, and shows that it practicable and feasible to do so.

Based on these conclusions, I would like to put forward the following recommendations for a systematic approach to altered pain processing (SATAPP.QST) for managing perioperative pain aiming to improve acute and chronic pain outcomes (summarised in Figure 16, below):

3.4.1 Clinical Implementation: Preoperative Period

Preoperatively, patients with a history suggestive of increased risk of poor pain outcomes (e.g. pre-existing chronic pain disorder; pre-existing chronic analgesic use, particularly opioids; extensive planned surgery; planned surgery with high risk of nerve damage or visceral pain; pain problems after previous surgery) should undergo screening quantitative sensory testing. This should include the flowing elements implemented in NASQ:

- testing for pain sensitivity using electric pain thresholds (skin) and pressure pain thresholds (deep tissues) close to and distant from the planned surgical incision
- testing for inhibitory pain modulation using the conditioned pain modulation paradigm involving electric skin and muscle pressure painful test stimulation and the cold pressor task as conditioning stimulation

If generalised heterotopic hyperalgesia suggestive of supraspinal central sensitisation is detected:

- Considerer treating this preoperatively, e.g. using gabapentinoids or ketamine infusion If poor inhibitory modulation is detected:
- Particular attention to intraoperative antinociception and antihyperalgesia is recommended, e.g. locoregional anaesthesia, ketamine infusion or nitrous oxide supplementation[202-205]
- Treatments possibly strengthening inhibitory controls should be considered, such as tricyclic antidepressants or other drugs affecting the monoaminergic systems (e.g. duloxitine[206])

The Effectiveness of therapeutic interventions should be monitored by subsequent serial NASQ measurements.

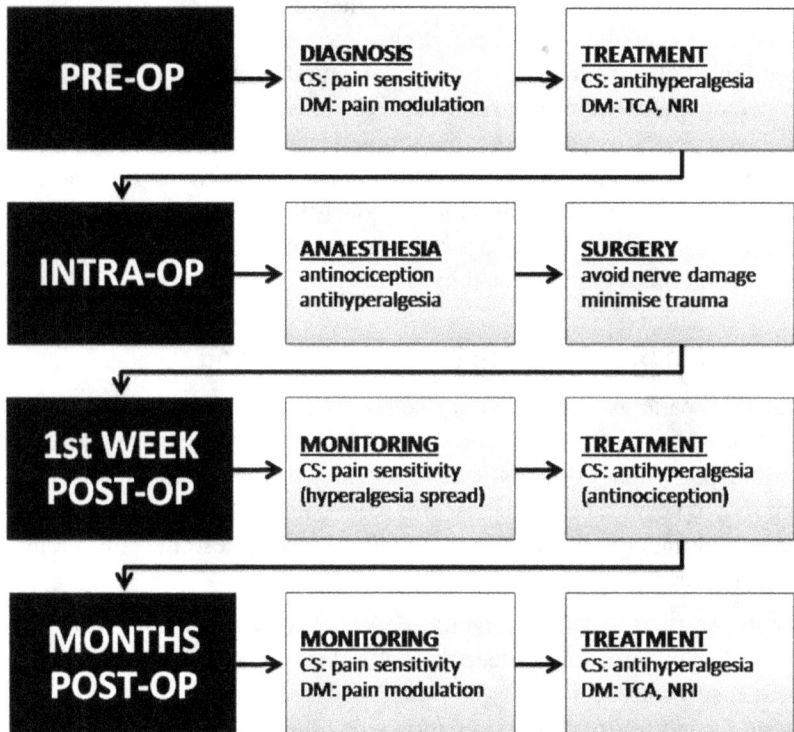

Figure 16   SATAPP.QST for perioperative pain management. CS = central sensitisation, DM=descending modulation, TCA = tricyclic antidepressants, NRI = noradrenaline reuptake inhibitors

3.4.2 Clinical Implementation: Intraoperative Period

Intraoperatively, patients with factors suggestive of increased risk of poor pain outcomes need special attention to reduce intraoperative sensitisation of their central nervous system, including the following measures:

- Anaesthetic techniques targeting effective antinociception, e.g. the use of loco-regional techniques continued into the postoperative period
- Use of medication limiting development of hyperalgesia, e.g. nitrous oxide or ketamine infusion extended into the postoperative period
- Application of surgical techniques avoiding/minimising nerve damage and limiting central sensitisation (local anaesthetic infiltration, reduced extensiveness of tissue damage via minimally invasive surgery)

3.4.3 Clinical Implementation: Early Postoperative Period

In the first postoperative week, patients need to be monitored using serial pain sensitivity measurements for development and persistence of spreading hyperalgesia, both nociception- and opioid-induced. This applies particularly to patients with factors suggestive of increased risk of poor pain outcomes. If hyperalgesia develops or persists, particularly of deep tissues such as muscle, the following should be considered:

- Institution/continuation of antihyperalgesic measures, e.g. ketamine infusion or gabapentinoids
- Starting treatments possibly strengthening inhibitory controls, e.g. tricyclic antidepressants or other drugs affecting the monoaminergic systems[206]
- Institution/continuation of effective antinociceptive measures, e.g. catheter local anaesthetic techniques

The effectiveness of therapeutic interventions should be monitored by serial NASQ measurements.

3.4.4 Clinical Implementation: Late Postoperative Period

During the subsequent postoperative period (months to year), patients at risk should:

- Continue to be monitored using serial pain sensitivity measurements for persistence and spread of hyperalgesia, particularly of deep tissues such as muscle
  If Hyperalgesia persists or spreads, consider:

- Institution/continuation of antihyperalgesic measures, e.g. gabapentinoids
- Dealing with ongoing nociceptive inputs, e.g. via long-term nerve blocks
- Also monitoring inhibitory function, e.g. via CPM paradigm, and starting treatments possibly strengthening inhibitory controls, e.g. tricyclic antidepressants or other drugs affecting the monoaminergic systems[206]

The effectiveness of therapeutic interventions should be monitored by serial NASQ measurements.

4

SATAPP.QST for Chronic Pain Practice

4.1 The Problem of Chronic Pain

4.1.1 Major Societal Impact

Chronic pain continues to be a costly and prevalent medical and societal problem with an estimated point prevalence of ca. 15–19% in Western societies[207,208]. About 35% of these patients report that the chronic pain significantly interferes with their daily activities of living[209]. The picture is even worse when considering treatment of chronic pain, where no treatment at present used eliminates pain for the majority of patients[210]. Thus, for example, use of anticonvulsants and antidepressants for chronic pain will achieve a 50% reduction in pain ratings in only one patient out of three[211]. The results of interventional treatments are even worse, e.g. between two thirds and three quarters of patients undergoing back surgery for pain will continue to experience pain for many years after surgery[212–214].

4.1.2 Symptom-based Approaches

This major problem facing pain medicine must be viewed in the context of the continuing symptom-based nature of our present diagnostic and therapeutic approaches to chronic pain. The history of medical progress suggests that most advances towards effective treatment are the result of better understanding and diagnostics of mechanisms underlying a given disease and its development[76,215]. Such understanding and diagnostics of pain diseases is largely lacking for the clinical chronic pain patients at present, and explains the poor therapeutic performance of pain medicine[76,198,215,216]. Thus the first and foremost challenge for clinical pain research is to understand the alterations in pain processing operating in patients with chronic pain, and to devise methods of diagnosing these in the clinical context.

4.1.3 Achieving SATAPP.QST

The basis for achieving a systematic approach to altered pain processing for chronic pain is an understanding of underlying changes in central pain processing. As previously mentioned, understanding and diagnosing altered central pain processing and its nature is key to answering *the four questions* regarding nociceptive processing in pain conditions, namely

1) Nociceptive source, 2) Nociceptive transmission, 3) Altered central pain processing and 4) Possible autonomy of altered central pain processing.

My research programme on chronic pain has focussed on questions three and four. Based on NASQ, I have concentrated on the diagnosis and quantification of spreading and generalised hyperalgesia as a manifestation of sensitised supraspinal pain processing, and its dependence on peripheral nociceptive drive (V, VII, VIII, IX, X, XIV, XV). I chose this topic as a continuation of my research programme on the relationship between the development of hyperalgesia and persistent pain after surgery.

As already discussed above, rostral neuraxial spread of central sensitisation manifest as spreading and generalised hyperalgesia seems to be a candidate process for the development of chronic pain[25–27]. Spreading or generalised hyperalgesia is now recognised as a feature of many chronic pain syndromes, being associated with extensive central excitation including supraspinal central sensitisation and cortical reorganisation as well as pro-nociceptive descending pain modulation states[25,26,33,35,43,49,60,61,66, 78,95,159,163].

Therapeutically, diagnosing generalised hyperalgesia as a marker for central sensitisation is important in the context of chronic pain because the underlying presence of central sensitisation means that treatments addressing peripheral nociceptive input alone are unlikely to be successful, likely requiring own specific, targeted therapeutic measures[187,197]. Taking these aspects together, there is a clear need to be able to validly and reliably diagnose spreading or generalised hyperalgesia in chronic pain patients – not only as a descriptor of the central sensitisation exhibited, but also as a marker of disease progression.

4.2 Summary of Current Knowledge: Neuroplasticity and Chronic Pain

4.2.1 Spreading Central Sensitisation of Nociceptive Processing

Evidence for the presence of generalized deep tissue hyperalgesia as a sign of supraspinal central sensitisation is now available in a large number of chronic pain conditions. In most cases this increased sensitivity to pain is demonstrated by psychophysical testing or QST, i.e. via pain magnitude ratings to standardized pain stimuli or via the determination of pain thresholds[51,52,55,56,67,68,79,91,217]. Using such methods, supraspinal central sensitization with chronic pain has now been demonstrated, e.g., in low back pain[45,57,176,177,194], fibromyalgia[44,46,48,80,105,109,160,218−222], rheumatoid arthritis[218,223,224], osteoarthritis[32,82,218,225], chronic widespread pain[48,219], irritable bowel syndrome[50,226,227], pancreatitis[228,229,] gallstones[230] and headache[181].

4.2.2 Pro-nociceptive Shifts in Pain Modulation

Further support for supraspinal alterations of pain processing is provided via evidence for loss of DNIC or descending facilitation using conditioned pain modulation (CPM) paradigms, e.g. involving the cold pressor task[112,231−233]. Evidence for such pro-nociceptive supraspinal modulation of pain processing accompanying chronic pain is available for a number of conditions including fibromyalgia[46,48,80,96,160,222,] muscle[94], headache[181], osteoarthritis[32,225], irritable bowel syndrome[50,227], and rheumatoid arthritis[223].

4.2.3 Sensitisation of Non-nociceptive Cortical Processing

In addition to mentioned signs of sensitized supraspinal pain processing, there is now increasing evidence for the presence of sensitisation of non-nociceptive supraspinal processing in the context of chronic pain disorders. Thus chronic low back pain has been linked to sensitized taste[234] and more extensive CRPS to sensitized hearing (hyperacusis)[235]. First evidence is now available showing alterations in affective and cognitive processing in chronic pain patients using a variety of cognitive function tests[29,78,149,221,236−238]. The application of modern neuroimaging (e.g. fMRI) and neuroelectro-physiological (e.g. source localization with multichannel EEG) techniques has made it possible to directly demonstrate cortical reorganization, altered connectivity and modulation associated with central sensitisation in asso-ciation with chronic pain conditions such as CRPS[49,239,240,] irritable bowel syndrome[227,] pancreatitis[241−246,] low back pain[78,163,236,247−249,] fibromyalgia[44,48,80,160,220−222,250−254,] and after amputation[255−259]. Indeed, it is not only specific non-nociceptive supraspinal processing which has been shown to be altered in chronic pain, there is now early data showing that even the global resting state of the brain is altered in chronic pain patients[149,248]. Furthermore, recent neuroimaging studies have demonstrated atrophy and brain substance loss in supratentorial structures to be present in a variety of chronic pain conditions[163,242,243,246,247,249].

There is thus now ample evidence that the chronic pain state is associated with supraspinal and supratentorial changes in brain processing, affecting not only nociceptive but also non-nociceptive processing. These changes are manifest as generalized hyperalgesia (particularly of deep tissues), alterations in non-nociceptive sensory processing, and the changes in cognitive, affective, mental or psychological function so characteristic of – and so well described in – chronic pain patients.

4.3 Synopsis of Own Contributions

4.3.1 Defining the Patients

In the course of my research, we chose four groups of patients with chronic pain of various aetiologies and durations, and affecting different tissues or systems. In the first instance, this choice was made in order to be able to study a wide variety of chronic pain patients. Equally important, this choice of patients also enabled the study of interesting and relevant other aspects of chronic pain, particularly 1) effects of disease duration and progression in relation to altered pain processing, and 2) relationships between peripheral nociceptive input and central alterations in pain processing. The patients groups I chose are briefly described in the following.

4.3.1.1 Neuroinflammatory pain: complex regional pain syndrome (CRPS) type I (vii)

We recruited patients diagnosed some eight years previously as having CRPS I according to the Veldman criteria 152, sub-diagnosis warm or cold, of a single upper extremity (V). All these patients had undergone a one-year standardised multidisciplinary therapy after diagnosis. Based on the answers to questioning, a disease progression score (DPS) was assigned to each patient: DPS $0 =$ no significant pain, no extension of CRPS to the other extremity; DPS $1 =$ significant pain, no extension; DPS $2 =$ significant pain and extension to another extremity. One of the major goals of this study was to define the relationship between progression of neuroinflammation and changes in central pain processing, e.g. the development of central sensitisation.

4.3.1.2 Combined somatic and neuropathic pain: low back pain (v)

The low back pain patients suffered from low back pain radiating into the leg with a duration of between one month and one year, and were now waiting for surgery of their prolapsed intervertebral disc. Their pain had been greater than visual analogue scale (VAS) 5 for more than three quarters of the time for at least one month, accompanied by typical symptoms and signs of sciatic pain. In addition they all had a significant intervertebral disc prolapse confirmed by neuroimaging. The indication for surgery was thus mainly based on pain, not on neurological impairment. All patients had furthermore undergone a (failed) trial of conservative treatment. Three days before surgery all were started on a standard anti-inflammatory regime of diclofenac 3 X 100 mg po. We studied all patients on the day before surgery under diclofenac treatment, some were pain-free under this regime, others not. The main emphasis of my research here was to study the impact of adding neuropathic pain to inflammatory somatic pain on the development of central sensitisation expressed as spreading hyperalgesia.

4.3.1.3 Viscero-somatic pain: chronic pancreatitis (viii, ix, xiv, xv)

Our group has generated a unique body of knowledge regarding central alterations in pain processing in chronic pancreatitis patients. For two studies (VIII, XIV), we recruited patients having suffered from severe pain due to chronic pancreatitis, mean duration 4–5 years, who were at present stable on opioid analgesic medication. None had experienced complications of chronic pancreatitis, undergone abdominal surgery, or suffered from other chronic pain syndromes. For comparison, we recruited a group of pain-free age- and gender-matched patients due to undergo minor, benign urological or gynaecological surgery as controls. The other two studies (IX, XV) included chronic pancreatitis patients scheduled for pain-relieving surgery, i.e. bilateral thoracoscopic splanchnicectomy (BTS). The indication for BTS was severe continuous or intermittent pancreatic pain necessitating continuous opioid medication for the last six months in combination with several unsuccessful attempts to reduce (or discontinue) opioid medication. At the time of preoperative measurement, these patients were stable on their opioid medication, none had complications of pancreatitis or other chronic pain syndromes. Patients' pain and pain processing were assessed before and ca. six weeks after BTS. Again we recruited a set of age- and gender-matched controls for comparison as necessary. This set of studies investigates 1) the effect of ongoing visceral nociceptive input on central sensitisation of somatic pain processing, 2) the effects on central somatic pain processing of deafferenting ongoing visceral nociceptive input, and 3) the effects of acute NMDA receptor blockade on the central sensitisation resulting from ongoing visceral nociceptive input.

4.3.1.4 Viscero-visceral pain: dysmenorrhoea

This study (X) recruited pre-menopausal women with significant dysmenorrhoea from a gynaecological outpatient's clinic. The patients suffered recurrent abdominal pain an average of eight years with a VAS intensity of over 60 mm related to the menstrual cycle, but were free of any other gastrointestinal symptoms or disorder, and did not suffer from any other pain disorder. For comparison, a matched health control group was recruited. All patients were measured mid-cycle to minimize effects of the menstrual cycle. The main aim of the study was to research whether ongoing visceral nociceptive input (e.g. due to dysmenorrhoea) results in sensitisation of convergent central visceral pain processing in other visceral structures (e.g. colon and rectum).

4.3.2 Characteristics of Altered Pain Processing in Chronic Pain Patients

All the chronic pain conditions we studied were accompanied by hyperalgesia, irrespective of duration and type of chronic pain studied, i.e. short and long-lasting; somatic, visceral and neuropathic. These results add to the growing body of clinical and experimental evidence linking chronic pain and hyperalgesia[32−34,45,46,50,105,142,150,176,260,261]. Our most consistent finding using NASQ was generalised hyperalgesia to pressure algometry; results using cutaneous electrical stimulation were more variable.

Pressure algometry results in stimulation of mechanoreceptors, mostly of deep tissues such as muscle, with only minor contributions from skin inputs[89,105,106]. It can therefore be considered to reflect changes in deep tissue pain processing, such as the mechanical hyperalgesia associated with central sensitisation[89,105,106]. Transcutaneous electrical stimulation, which reflects mainly pain processing originating from the skin, bypasses skin nociceptors, stimulating the nociceptive nerve afferents directly[108,109]. Electric thresholds thus effectively reflect more central changes in cutaneous pain processing, being sensitive to both excitatory (e.g. central sensitisation) and inhibitory (e.g. DNIC) changes[46,107−109].

My studies link chronic pain syndromes to spreading or generalised heterotopic hyperalgesia which is mechanical and affects deep somatic tissues, in our case muscle, in keeping with the literature regarding chronic pain[32,45,50,105,176,260]. The presence of spreading or generalised hyperalgesia in these patients is compatible with a variety of possible underlying pathophysiological processes: *Firstly*, it may indicate that central sensitisation is spreading rostrally up the neuraxis to involve supraspinal structures[30,31,142,150]. *Secondly*, this pattern of hyperalgesia might be a reflection of the involvement of perispinal macroglia, which can be sensitised by humoral as well as neuronal mechanisms[262,263]. A *third* possible cause for generalised hyperalgesia in chronic pain patients is opioid-induced hyperalgesia, which shares many of the same mechanisms as nociception-induced hyperalgesia. This typically accompanies longer-term, escalating, use of potent opioids – which is typical for many chronic pain conditions, and is now well-described in the literature in the animal experimental as well as human clinical context[27,111,264−269].

The reality of the *first*-mentioned mechanism in chronic pain patients is now well-demonstrated by human clinical studies using advanced neurodiagnostic and neuroimaging techniques[49,78,159,163,236,239]. The *second* mechanism is well-documented experimentally[262,263,270−273] but awaits similar clinical confirmation. The *third* mechanism, opioid-induced hyperalgesia, is also quite well studied experimentally. It has also been demonstrated in human volunteers and humans[111,264,274−276]. Once these processes have persisted for longer periods of time, they may become progressively more difficult to reverse and increasingly involve architectural as opposed to purely functional changes, with the accompanying hyperalgesia thus becoming gradually more autonomous, i.e. less dependent on the original peripheral nociceptive inputs[25,161,162,270]. The postulated course of events is summarised in Figure 17, below.

The effects of chronic pain on skin electric pain processing were more variable than on pressure algometry. Acute pain typically results in descending inhibitory modulation to the skin – if this inhibitory system is intact, which may not always the case in chronic pain patients[35,46,230,244]. The fact that in our study of low back pain patients (V), acute sciatica was related to higher pain thresholds suggests that in these relatively short-duration chronic pain patients, descending inhibitory modulation was still intact, although we did not formally test this, e.g. using the CPM paradigm. The presence of deep tissue hyperalgesia does not appear to necessarily translate into skin hyperalgesia. For example, for the chronic pancreatitis pain of visceral origin, skin hyperalgesia seems to be the exception rather than the rule, as also described by others for

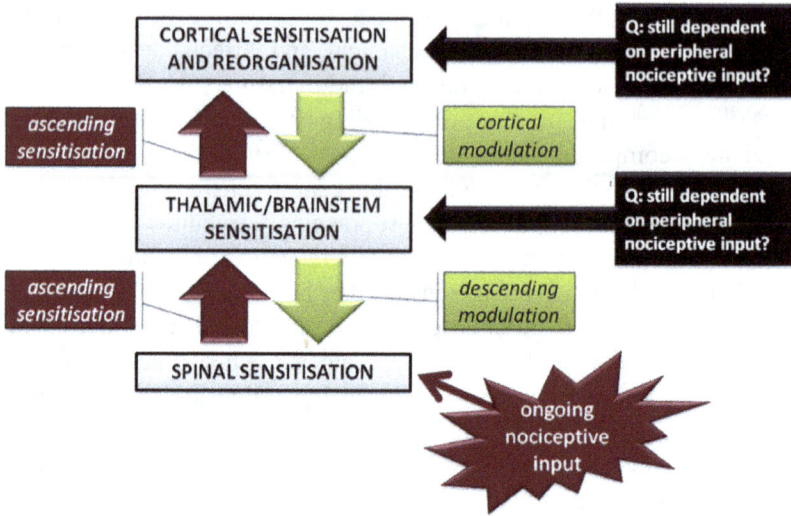

Figure 17   This schematic illustrates the concept of neuraxial proliferation of central sensitisation as the basis for development of generalised hyperalgesia in chronic pain. Each stage of rostral spread of central sensitisation is subject to descending modulatory control from superior segments; if descending inhibitory control is inadequate further rostral spread of sensitisation occurs. Note that modulation can be either inhibitory or facilitatory. A central question in chronic pain is whether the central sensitisation present is still dependent for its persistence on ongoing caudal nociceptive inputs

visceral pain[230,260]. On the other hand, in both low back pain patients (which have generalised muscle hyperalgesia[45]) and "cold" CRPS I patients (which also exhibit muscle hyperalgesia[277]), some form of generalised cutaneous hyperalgesia to electrical stimulation was present in our studies (V, VII).

My studies provide evidence that central sensitisation spreads in the neuraxis with ongoing nociceptive input, a process expressed as the phenomenon of spreading hyperalgesia. This spread can *firstly* be heterotopic within somatic tissues, e.g. somato-somatic spread from muscle to skin, as seen in low back pain, CRPS or chronic pain after surgery. As seen in the CRPS patients, this spread seems to be related to disease progression. *Secondly*, viscero-visceral spread of central sensitisation is equally possible, as illustrated by the dysmenorrhoea study with spread of hyperalgesia from gynaecological to intestinal viscera. *Finally*, this spread may even be viscero-somatic, as seen in the chronic pancreatitis patients with their hyperalgesia to muscle stimulation.

We would therefore suggest that the persistence and spread of hyperalgesia should be considered diagnostically characteristic of chronic pain. Heterotopic spread of hyperalgesia, particularly to deep tissues, appears to be associated with more severe pain disorder in this context. Thus the diagnosis and quantification of spreading or generalised heterotopic hyperalgesia appears to be of key importance in chronic pain, because its presence signals the existence of prognostically serious alterations in pain processing. Also seen in the context of chronic pain persistence after surgery[178] (XIII), these alterations risk becoming progressively more difficult to influence by measures blocking peripheral nociceptive inputs – and thus increasingly difficult to influence or reverse. Diagnosing such hyperalgesia provides the basis for specific treatment targeting central sensitisation, pro-nociceptive shifts in central pain modulation and allied changes to the central nervous system in chronic pain patients, mechanisms frequently only inadequately addressed by current conventional treatment regimes.

4.3.3 Disease Progression and Diagnostic Subgroups

Not only does generalised hyperalgesia accompany chronic pain syndromes, it also seems that the degree of spreading or generalised hyperalgesia may be linked to the progression of chronic pain syndromes. I specifically tested this hypothesis in our CRPS study (VII), confirming that, eighth years after original diagnosis, the degree of muscle pressure hyperalgesia was increased with increasing disease progression (as defined by extension to other extremities), as also suggested by other authors for CRPS and hyperalgesia[49,239,278,279]. I further found that hyperalgesia measured by pressure algometry was consistently greatest in the originally affected extremity.

Although both "warm" and "cold" CRPS I exhibited muscle hyperalgesia, these findings were more pronounced in diagnostic subgroup "cold" CRPS patients. These same "cold" CRPS patients also had worse clinical pain outcomes eight years after original diagnosis. Only in this group did degree of pressure hyperalgesia significantly correlate with clinical pain outcome measures. Interestingly, hyperalgesia to suprathreshold electrical skin stimulation was seen only in the "cold" diagnostic subgroup – and occurred in the absence of shifts in electric skin pain thresholds. Furthermore, this hyperalgesia was also linked to disease progression (Figure 18, below). Suprathreshold hyperalgesia is considered to be more reflective of sensitisation of supraspinal pain processing than hyperalgesia at threshold[29]. These findings support the hypothesis that central sensitisation is more severe and extensive in patients diagnosed with "cold" CRPS. They further suggest that in "cold" CRPS I patients, extensive rostral neuraxial progression of central sensitisation of pain

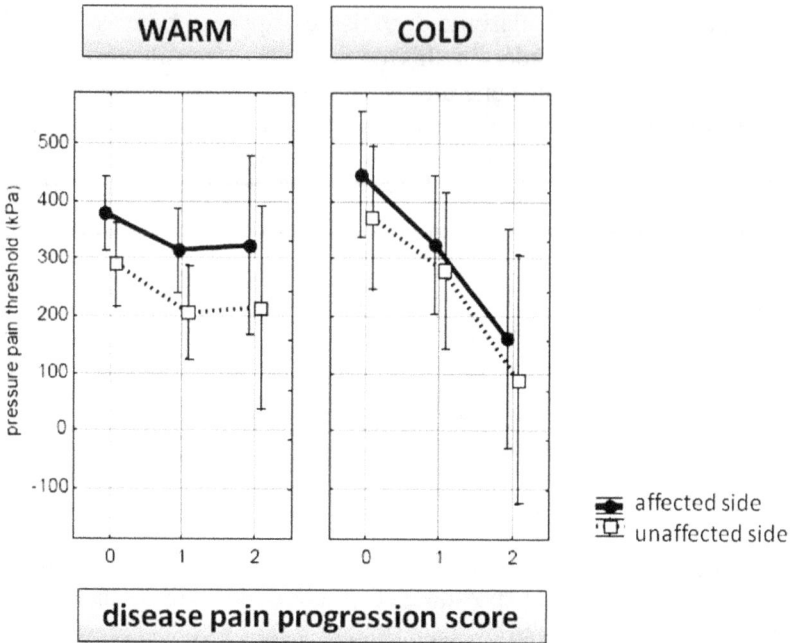

Figure 18   Pressure pain thresholds (in kPa; means and 95% confidence intervals) in CRPS I patients were significantly lower on the affected (vs. unaffected) side. They were also lower with increasing disease progression (DPPS). DIAG, original diagnosis (i.e. warm or cold CRPS 1); DPPS, disease pain progression score (0, no significant pain; 1, significant pain only in affected extremity; 2, significant pain in affected extremity plus extension to other extremity). Modified after dissertation reference VII

processing, linked to disease progression as well as poorer clinical outcome, has taken place. This appears not to be the case for "warm" CRPS patients, even eight years after diagnosis, where central sensitisation does not explain disease progression or clinical outcome. Thus rostral neuraxial progression of central sensitisation would appear to be a major underlying mechanism in "cold" CRPS I patients, while other mechanisms would appear to be operating in "warm" CRPS I patients.

Our results regarding the presence of central sensitisation in CRPS I patients are well-supported by an extensive body of literature using both QST and neurodiagnostic techniques to demonstrate central sensitisation and cortical reorganisation[49,239,240,277,280]. However, these studies neither differentiate between diagnostic subtypes, nor provide a link with disease progression, nor demonstrate the conjunction of deep tissue threshold hyperalgesia with cutaneous suprathreshold hyperalgesia seen in our study for "cold" CRPS I.

We conclude that 1) more severe and extensive hyperalgesia, particularly of muscle, is related to greater disease progression in CRPS I, and 2) "cold" (vs. "warm") CRPS I patients have signs of more prominent and extensive central sensitisation associated with a worse clinical prognosis. Interestingly, this intuitively attractive concept of a relationship between disease progression, disease subtypes and extent/severity of central sensitisation has not yet been applied to other clinical pain syndromes to date, and awaits further formal studies.

QST diagnostics regarding presence, degree, extent and modality patterns of hyperalgesia would appear to have realistic and useful potential to clinically quantify disease progression in the context of chronic pain syndromes. Furthermore, QST makes possible first attempts at mechanism-based diagnostic categorisation of chronic pain syndromes as a basis for more rational and effective treatment approaches, e.g. targeted specifically at the management of central sensitisation as opposed to conventional therapy directed at nociceptive inputs.

4.3.4 Gender Effects

The healthy control subjects in our chronic pancreatitis studies showed characteristic gender-related differences in pain processing. As reported in the literature, men had significantly higher pressure pain tolerance thresholds than women, without significant differences in pain sensitivity to electric stimulation[107,108,281]. The same pattern of lower pressure pain thresholds in women was also seen the pancreatitis patients. Interestingly, on reanalysis of our CRPS study (unpublished, reanalysis of VII), increased pain sensitivity in females was found not only for pressure pain thresholds, but also for electrically evoked pain in patients with the more serious, "cold" form of CRPS (Figure 19, below).

The results showing quite different responses regarding central pain processing of men vs. women to the chronic visceral nociceptive input of chronic pancreatitis are entirely novel, and were restricted to the study involving pancreatitis patients not having undergone previous abdominal surgery. Thus men appear to respond to chronic visceral nociceptive input by developing generalised somatic deep tissue hyperalgesia. Women do not develop such generalised hyperalgesia (at least not to the same degree), instead they exhibit localised hypoalgesia to electric skin stimulation in the referred pancreatic

Current effect: F(2, 86)=5,8165, p=,00427

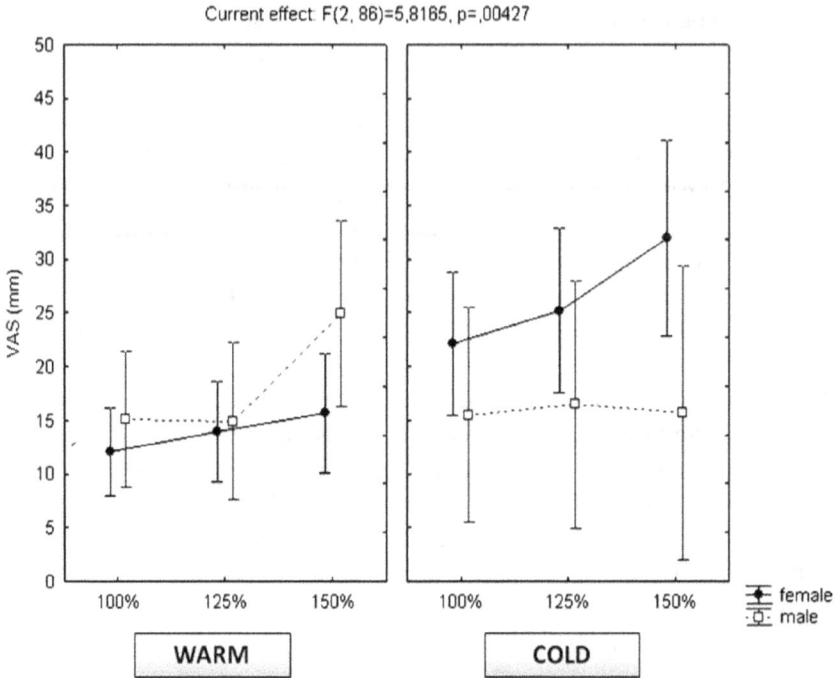

Figure 19   For "cold" CRPS 1 patients, electrically evoked pain (VAS in mm; means and 95% confidence intervals; at 100%, 125% and 150% of pain threshold) was significantly higher in females. DIAGN, original CRPS diagnosis (i.e. warm or cold). Reanalysis of results from study VII

dermatome. This is consistent with a segmental inhibitory response, which appears effective in limiting the development of generalised deep tissue hyperalgesia.

There are thus fundamental gender differences in the consequences of ongoing pancreatic nociceptive input regarding pain processing. While there are some reports detailing differences in pain processing between men and women, these mainly concern differences in pain sensitivity, often connected with the menstrual cycle[67,68,107,108,276,281−285]. Gender differences in the response to ongoing nociceptive input and its modulation are only sparsely described in the literature to date, particularly in the human, clinical context. Human gender differences have been reported concerning stress-induced analgesia as well as supraspinal descending noxious inhibitory control (DNIC) mechanisms[96,284,286], but we have found no mention of gender differences in segmental inhibitory mechanisms. These differences might be related to specific adaptations of female pain processing to the pain associated with childbirth. However, there is no literature available in this area at present, and further research is clearly indicated in this field.

The importance of diagnosing gender differences regarding alterations in pain processing in chronic pain diseases using QST is evident, because such diagnosis provides the necessary basis for subsequent treatment approaches targeting altered pain processing.

4.3.5 Effects of Antihyperalgesic Treatment

If central sensitisation manifest as heterotopic spreading hyperalgesia is a key mechanism in chronic pain, then it would be important to define and validate effective treatments for this condition. It is known that the NMDA receptor plays an important role in the development of central sensitisation, and NMDA receptor blockade has been experimentally demonstrated to inhibit central sensitisation[188,197,199,287−292]. Ketamine is a clinically available NMDA receptor blocker, and has been shown to improve pain outcomes after surgery[37,40,187,190−192,293,294] – and to reduce opioid-induced hyperalgesia when used perioperatively[186,295]. My study is the first to demonstrate the targeted use of a short-term infusion of ketamine to achieve acute inhibition of heterotopic spreading hyperalgesia in chronic pancreatitis patients with severe pain (Figure 20, below) (XIV). However, the infusion duration was too short to achieve significant decreases in clinical pain experience, illustrating the urgent need for further research in this field involving longer-term treatment approaches. The promise of pursuing such approaches targeting altered pain processing in severe chronic pain syndromes such as chronic pancreatitis is supported by a recent companion publication from our group, demonstrating the analgesic efficacy of another central antihyperalgesic agent, pregabalin, in relieving the pain of chronic pancreatitis[296]. Taken together, these results further underline the usefulness of QST in the management of chronic pain, not only in achieving a choice of pharmacological agent based on effects on pain processing, but also by providing a means of monitoring treatment effect and response.

4.3.6 Effects of Nociceptive Deafferentation

One of the key questions regarding the spreading hyperalgesia accompanying chronic pain syndromes is how dependent is the supraspinal central sensitisation which it reflects on ongoing nociceptive input for its maintenance[161,162].

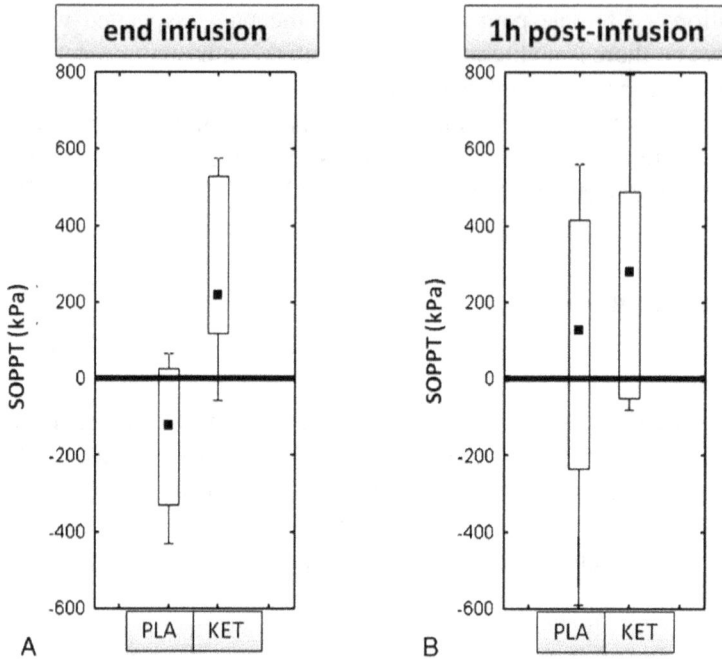

Figure 20 **A**. The change in sum of pressure pain thresholds (SOPPT, in kPa) immediately after the end of infusion versus before infusion of the trial medication compared for the placebo and S-ketamine groups. **B**. The change in SOPPT versus before infusion 1 hr after the end of infusion of the trial medication compared for the placebo and S-ketamine groups. The difference between groups immediately after the end of the infusion is significant – but not 1 hour later. Modified after dissertation reference XIV

The clinical use of bilateral thoracoscopic splanchnicectomy (BTS), an operation effectively leading to sensory denervation of the pancreas as a means of treating otherwise intractable pain accompanying chronic pancreatitis[297,298], provides an interesting opportunity to study the dependence of spreading hyperalgesia on ongoing nociceptive inputs. We studied this phenomenon in two groups of chronic pancreatitis patients undergoing BTS for chronic intractable pain.

In the first study BTS resulted in cessation of opioid therapy in about half the patients, who also showed a trend towards lower pain scores. There was, on average, a generalised increase in both deep tissue mechanical and cutaneous electric pain thresholds 6 weeks after BTS, suggesting that the supraspinal central sensitisation present in these patients is at least partially dependent on pancreatic nociceptive inputs. Male chronic pancreatitis patients underwent reversal of their generalised pressure hyperalgesia with BTS, while women showed increased segmental inhibition, particularly in those reporting clinical treatment success. At the time, we explained our heterogeneous findings in part by our choice of a relatively insensitive clinical pain endpoint. Further possible explanations included the presence in some patients of autonomous central sensitisation (i.e. independent of nociceptive input[161,162]), incomplete nociceptive deafferentation (e.g. due to surgical failure or because of ongoing pancreatic nociceptive input to the central nervous system via humoral mediators such as cytokines or interleukins[262,263,272,299]), or the act of deafferentation itself causing additional central sensitisation[25,31,257−259,290,300].

We studied BTS effects on central pain processing and its relation to clinical pain experience in more detail in the second study. Overall I demonstrated a negative correlation between change in pain VAS and change in pressure pain thresholds after BTS. A key finding was that patients where BTS resulted in a decrease in spreading hyperalgesia also showed a significant reduction in pain VAS. Patients where BTS caused no decrease (or even increase) in hyperalgesia showed no significant pain reduction (Figure 21, below). Interestingly, no such relation could be demonstrated for pancreatic segment hyperalgesia. These results suggest that in one group of pancreatitis patients treated by BTS (ca. 60%), central sensitisation expressed as spreading hyperalgesia is still dependent on peripheral nociceptive drive, and thus deafferentation by BTS results in pain reduction. In the other group (ca. 40%), central sensitisation has become independent of peripheral drive, thus deafferentation via BTS neither reduces hyperalgesia nor decreases pain.

We have found only one report in the literature addressing the question of reversibility of central sensitisation, and its dependence on ongoing nociceptive input[32]. This study demonstrated generalised deep tissue hyperalgesia to pressure algometry in patients with painful chronic osteoarthritis of the hip joint. The hyperalgesia (and the accompanying deficit of descending inhibitory modulation) was no longer present 6 months after endoprosthetic hip surgery rendering the patient pain-free. For the chronic osteoarthritis patients studied, this strongly suggests that central sensitisation and accompanying generalised hyperalgesia are reversible and dependent on ongoing nociceptive input for their maintenance.

The question of whether or not central sensitisation and its accompanying spreading hyperalgesia have progressed to a stage where they are autonomous and no longer dependent on ongoing nociceptive input is crucial for the choice of treatment approaches for chronic pain syndromes – and for the prediction of

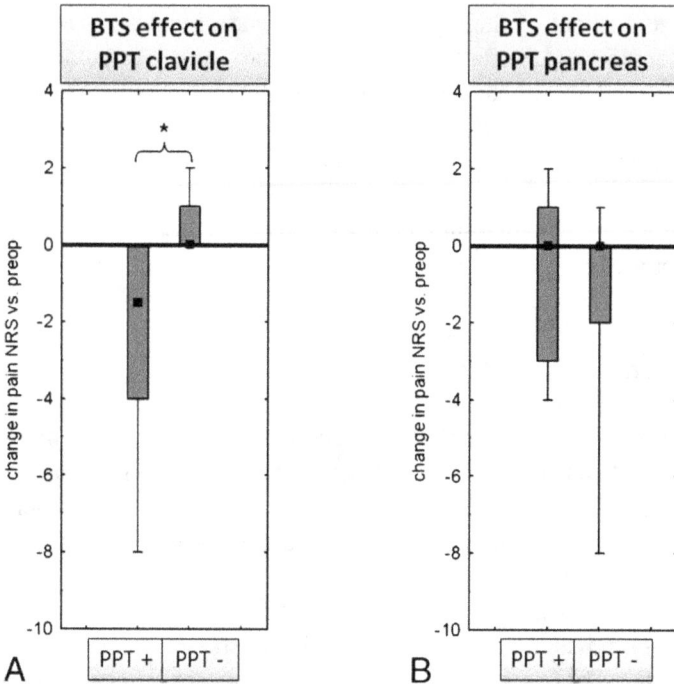

Figure 21   Box plots of change in pain numeric rating scores (NRS) vs. direction of change in pressure pain thresholds (PPT) after BTS. PPT was measured in the clavicle and pancreas dermatomes. **A.** The change in pain NRS after BTS was significantly greater (marked with an asterisk) in PPT + patients (hypoalgesic vs. preop) in the clavicle site after BTS. **B.** This was not the case for the pancreatic site. The PPT + (hypoalgesic) group experienced an increase in PPT after BTS (i.e. a reduction in preoperative hyperalgesia), the PPT- (hyperalgesic) group was the group not experiencing such an increase. Modified after dissertation reference XV

treatment outcomes. The identification of patients where central sensitisation has become autonomous is key, as in these patients techniques based on nociceptive deafferentation, e.g. opioids or nerve blocking techniques – are unlikely to be effective, and techniques targeting central pain processing are indicated. Our research is the first to identify this phenomenon as a mechanism present in therapeutic non-responders and further underlines the central role of QST for hyperalgesia diagnosis and monitoring. Clearly, further research is necessary in this area.

4.4 Summary: SATAPP.QST and Chronic Pain

In summary, my research into altered pain processing using NASQ in chronic pain patients has identified spreading, heterotopic hyperalgesia, particularly of deep tissues, as a constant and characteristic feature of chronic pain. Its presence suggests that the body has not succeeded in restricting central sensitisation due to ongoing nociceptive inputs to the spinal cord, and that central sensitisation may have progressed rostrally up the neuraxis to include supraspinal structures. Such deep tissue hyperalgesia appears to occur irrespective of the type of chronic pain syndrome under consideration, and to become visible early on in development, i.e. within months of start of pain.

Thus we would suggest that the presence of **spreading deep tissue hyperalgesia** be considered a basic criterion for the diagnosis of established chronic pain syndrome.

4.4.1 Relevance for Clinical Use

To my knowledge, this is the first time hyperalgesia characteristics of chronic pain have been investigated systematically. Based on my research, the following conclusions can be drawn:

Firstly, hyperalgesia spread in chronic pain is typically heterotopic, and can be somato-somatic, viscero-somatic and viscero-visceral. There is considerable inter-individual variation of onset/vulnerability to hyperalgesia and its spread, only individually diagnosable using QST.

Secondly, hyperalgesia spread is associated with clinical progression of chronic pain. Differences in characteristics of hyperalgesia spread may be associated with differences in disease subtype, e.g. warm vs. cold CRPS I. This underlines the diagnostic, prognostic and therapeutic relevance of monitoring of hyperalgesia spread using QST.

Thirdly, there are significant differences associated with gender in basal pain sensitivity, the dynamics of hyperalgesia development and response of hyperalgesia to treatment in the context of chronic pain disorders. These differences are only visible using QST.

Fourthly, central sensitisation manifest as spreading hyperalgesia can become independent of peripheral nociceptive inputs, and thus no longer respond to treatments based on peripheral deafferentation such as nerve blocks or opioids. We are the first to formally documented this phenomenon. It has important therapeutic implications, i.e. the targeted use of drugs acting on central sensitisation, and can only be diagnosed/monitored using QST.

Fifthly, correlations between clinical pain measures and QST measures of hyperalgesia were either absent or variable. QST and clinical pain measures thus provide different but complementary information. For chronic as for perioperative pain, QST is needed to diagnose presence/spread of hyperalgesia as a sign of rostral spread of central sensitisation.

Sixthly, spreading hyperalgesia as a manifestation of central sensitisation can be inhibited by specific treatments, such as the NMDA receptor antagonist ketamine. These therapeutic effects can only be documented and monitored using QST techniques.

Finally, implementation of these conclusions in clinical chronic pain practice is impossible without implementing QST diagnostics. Our QST research has not only shown the usefulness of NASQ in clinical chronic pain practice, it has also proven the practicability of SATAPP.QST.

4.4.2 Clinical Implementation

Our conclusions above show that clinical implementation of SATAPP.QST requires QST diagnostics, validated and implemented in the NASQ paradigm with the following features:

- Multimodal test stimulation, electrical and mechanical stimulation are sensitive to secondary hyperalgesia/central sensitisation; electric skin stimulation is sensitive to inhibitory modulation, and pressure algometry detects deep tissue hyperalgesia.
- Multi-site test stimulation, to detect and define spreading hyperalgesia. As a minimum, sites close to/distant from the painful area should be tested.
- Test stimulation repeated in time, to document the time course of altered pain processing and its relation to chronic pain development and progression.
- Static and dynamic QST paradigms. Static QST tests passive basal pain sensitivity (e.g. hyperalgesia); dynamic QST uses conditioning painful stimulation to test how the body actively modulates nociceptive input (e.g. CPM/DNIC paradigm).

My recommendations for the clinical implementation using NASQ for SATAPP.QST in the management of chronic pain disorders are summarised in the diagramme below (Figure 22).

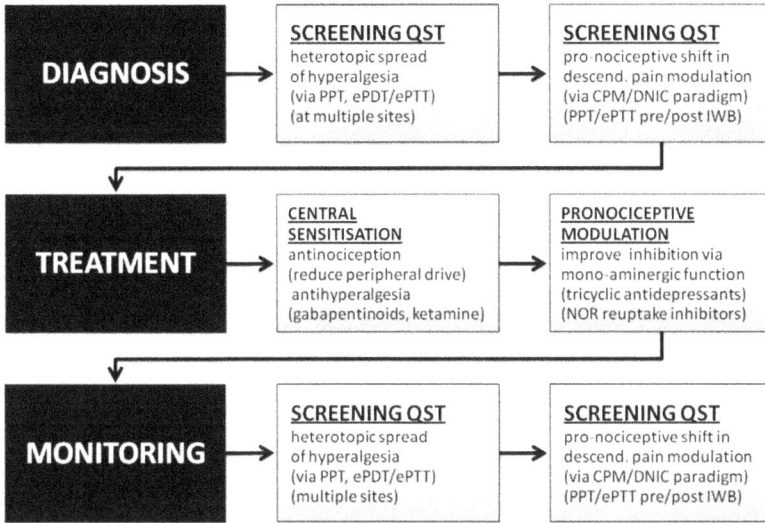

Figure 22 SATAPP.QST in chronic pain disorders. PPT = pressure pain threshold, ePDT = electric pain detection threshold, ePTT = electric pain tolerance threshold, CPM = conditioned pain modulation paradigm, DNIC = diffuse noxious inhibitory controls, NRI = noradrenaline reuptake inhibitor

5

SATAPP.QST for Pain Medicine: Conclusions

5.1 NASQ: The Basis for SATAPP.QST for Pain Medicine

My research has shown spreading, heterotopic hyperalgesia, likely an expression of rostrally spreading central sensitisation, to be the key alteration in pain processing associated with chronic pain and its development. This phenomenon is linked to pro-nociceptive shifts in endogenous (descending) pain modulation. Based on the Nijmegen-Aalborg Screening QST (NASQ) paradigm we developed, I have demonstrated the feasibility and usefulness of using quantitative sensory testing (QST) to diagnose and monitor characteristic changes in pain processing accompanying development, progression and presence of chronic pain. This demonstration makes implementation of a systematic approach to altered pain processing in clinical practice feasible – and urgently desirable. My work has shown this paradigm shift to be attainable for both perioperative and chronic pain practice.

My research has defined a QST paradigm (the Nijmegen-Aalborg Screening QST, NASQ) suitable for a systematic approach to altered pain processing (SATAPP.QST). The NASQ paradigm includes at least two measurement points (close to/distant from painful site), two stimulation modalities (electric and pressure stimulation) and a CPM paradigm (cold pressor task as conditioning stimulation). It is well-accepted by all patients and can be completed in about 30 minutes. The NASQ-based research presented does not cover specific QST diagnostics for neuropathic pain, where thermal QST appears particularly useful for the diagnosis of peripheral nerve damage[67,68,194]. My systematic approach to managing chronic pain and its development (Figure 23, below) as the basis for effective prognosis, diagnosis, prevention and treatment of pain disorders, is summarised below (Figure 23).

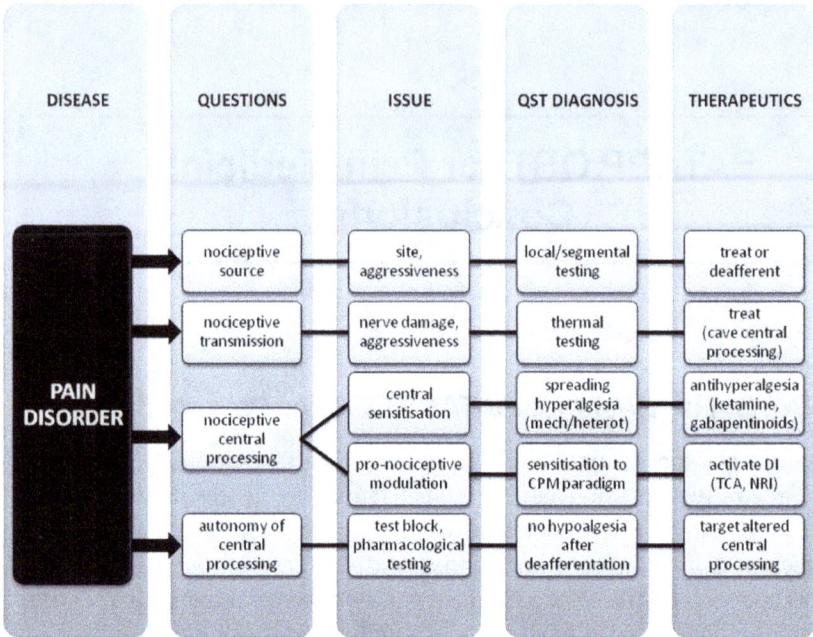

Figure 23   Schematic for a systematic approach to altered pain processing (SATAPP.QST) using QST (NASQ) for pain medicine. Autonomy means that alterations in central pain processing (e.g. central sensitisation) have become independent of peripheral nociceptive drive. Mech = mechanical, heterot = heterotopic, CPM = conditioned pain modulation, DI = descending inhibition, TCA = tricyclic antidepressants, NRI = noradrenaline reuptake inhibitors

5.2 SATAPP.QST and Perioperative Pain

In the *perioperative* context, I have for the first time been able to demonstrate that poorer preoperative endogenous pain modulation is associated with a greater risk of persistence and spread of postoperative hyperalgesia as well as a greater chance of having chronic pain six months after surgery. We further showed that patients ultimately reporting chronic pain at six months after surgery show a characteristic pattern of postoperative persistence and spread of heterotopic hyperalgesia. Such postoperative hyperalgesia is sensitive to both antinociceptive (nerve block, opioids) and antihyperalgesic (ketamine) interventions. These perioperative insights were gained using our simple NASQ paradigm lasting maximally 30 minutes, involving at least two measurement sites (close to and distant from surgery), two types of stimulation (electric, pressure) and a CPM paradigm involving cold pressor task.

Our results suggest the usefulness and feasibility of perioperative QST monitoring using NASQ for achieving a rational and effective systematic approach to altered pain processing in the context of 1) preoperative assessment for risk of chronic pain after surgery, 2) postoperative monitoring for early signs of chronic pain development, and 3) monitoring of effectiveness of perioperative management regarding chronic pain prevention and treatment. SATAPP.QST based on NASQ brings with it the realistic promise of significant improvements in surgical pain outcomes. Furthermore, it should also provide the basis for making perioperative pain management tangibly more effective – and resource-efficient – in the foreseeable future.

5.3 SATAPP.QST and Chronic Pain

For *chronic pain* patients, I have shown that spreading hyperalgesia made visible using NASQ is ubiquitous to a variety of chronic pain syndromes at various stages of progression. I was for the first able to systematically establish how the characteristics of spreading hyperalgesia are influenced by disease progression, disease subtype and gender, making these characteristics useful for process-oriented approaches to disease diagnosis and prognosis as well as for determining indications for specific disease treatments. In particular, we were able to demonstrate that specific treatment for central sensitisation (e.g. ketamine) inhibited its manifestation as hyperalgesia, and that this effect could be monitored using our NASQ paradigm. Furthermore, I was for the first time able to specifically demonstrate that in certain chronic pain patients, central changes in pain processing have become autonomous, i.e. independent of peripheral nociceptive drive. These findings are crucial because they carry the message that in certain chronic pain patients, nociceptive deafferentation (e.g. nerve blocks, opioids) will be therapeutically ineffective – and that treatment targeting altered central processing is the key to successful management.

Again these insights regarding chronic pain were gained using our simple NASQ paradigm. Not lasting more than 30 minutes, the NASQ paradigm involves several measurement sites at variable distances from pain to determine hyperalgesia topography, at least two types of stimulation (electric, pressure) and a CPM paradigm involving cold pressor task. Our findings confirm the usefulness and feasibility of SATAPP.QST using NASQ for chronic pain management. This ap proach forms the basis of rational and effective systematic approaches to altered pain processing as the basis for 1) diagnosis and prognosis of chronic pain, including subtype definition,

2) monitoring for signs of chronic pain progression, 3) making a rational choice of treatment option with a view to maximising treatment response, and 4) ongoing monitoring of effectiveness of chronic pain treatment and management.

Consequently applied to the clinical practice of chronic pain, introduction of SATAPP.QST and NASQ should not only make the diagnostics of chronic pain much more effective and reliable, it also carries the potential to greatly reduce the cost and burden of chronic pain treatment by making achievement of therapeutic response more rapid and predictable in the individual patient.

5.4 Implementing SATAPP.QST: Aim of the Present Review

The present review provides not only the initial basis, but also the much-needed impetus for the urgently necessary paradigm shift in pain medicine away from symptom-based management towards a systematic approach to altered pain processing in pain diseases. To this end, we have now provided data substantiating three central concepts, namely:

1) Quantitative sensory testing to make visible altered pain process-ing, implemented via the simple NASQ paradigm, represents a valid diagnostic method suitable for achieving SATAPP in routine clinical practice;
2) Implementation of SATAPP by applying NASQ provides real clinical benefit in the diagnostics, prognostics and monitoring of chronic pain disorders and their progression; and
3) First evidence is now available that pain management paradigms based on SATAPP and NASQ are therapeutically feasible and successful when applied in everyday clinical practice.

Based on the research I have done over the last fifteen years, we have now provided a first foundation for the implementation of systematic approach to altered pain processing in everyday clinical pain practice in the very near future. Taken together, the three statements listed above demonstrate not only the feasibility, but also the necessity of now urgently addressing the task of implementing a systematic approach to altered pain processing (SATAPP.QST) to achieve long-awaited and necessary improvement in everyday clinical practice of pain diagnostics and therapeutics.

5.5 SATAPP.QST: Future Perspectives

Based on our development of a standardised and validated clinical approach (SATAPP.QST), *large-scale clinical studies* defining the presence and pattern of altered pain processing in groups of patients suffering from defined chronic pain syndromes using standardised diagnostics (NASQ) are the next necessary step. These studies should investigate not only hyperalgesia and its characteristics, but also the nature and effectiveness of the inhibitory responses mounted by the body. In order to be able to diagnose hyperalgesia and pro-nociceptive shifts in pain modulation, normal subjects should be studied to generate normal values for pain processing. The large-scale nature of these studies is necessary due to the large variability in the nervous system response to ongoing nociceptive input regarding both sensitisation and subsequent modulation.

Apart from the characterisation of the role of generalised hyperalgesia in chronic pain, other allied topics also need investigating, including how hyperalgesia develops and changes over time as the pain disease progresses, the question of if and when supraspinal central sensitisation becomes independent from ongoing nociceptive input, and the impact of gender on the pain processing and inhibition in chronic pain. At a later stage, these studies need to include systematic study of therapeutic interventions, defining their effects on pain processing in health and disease using NASQ, as the basis for developing rational approaches to chronic pain management systematically targeting altered pain processing. Furthermore, it would be useful to be able to develop further QST parameters predictive of ultimate disease outcome and treatment response of chronic pain disorders, to permit targeting of medical resources at patients with greatest risk of poor outcomes.

References

1. Lynch EP, Lazor MA, Gellis JE, Orav J, Goldman L, Marcantonio ER: Patient experience of pain after elective noncardiac surgery. Anesth Analg 1997; 85: 117–23
2. Svensson I, Sjostrom B, Haljamae H: Assessment of pain experiences after elective surgery. J Pain Symptom Manage 2000; 20: 193–201
3. Dolin SJ, Cashman JN, Bland JM: Effectiveness of acute postoperative pain management: I. Evidence from published data. Br J Anaesth 2002; 89: 409–23
4. Pogatzki-Zahn EM, Zahn PK, Brennan TJ: Postoperative pain–clinical implications of basic research. Best Pract Res Clin Anaesthesiol 2007; 21: 3–13
5. Apfelbaum JL, Chen C, Mehta SS, Gan TJ: Postoperative pain experience: results from a national survey suggest postoperative pain continues to be undermanaged. Anesth Analg 2003; 97: 534–40, table of contents
6. Perkins FM, Kehlet H: Chronic pain as an outcome of surgery. A review of predictive factors. Anesthesiology 2000; 93: 1123–33
7. Macrae WA: Chronic pain after surgery. Br J Anaesth 2001; 87: 88–98
8. Kehlet H, Jensen TS, Woolf CJ: Persistent postsurgical pain: risk factors and prevention. Lancet 2006; 367: 1618–25
9. Callesen T: Inguinal hernia repair: anaesthesia, pain and convalescence. Dan Med Bull 2003; 50: 203–18
10. Mikkelsen T, Werner MU, Lassen B, Kehlet H: Pain and sensory dysfunction 6 to 12 months after inguinal herniotomy. Anesth Analg 2004; 99: 146–51
11. Aasvang E, Kehlet H: Chronic postoperative pain: the case of inguinal herniorrhaphy. Br J Anaesth 2005; 95: 69–76
12. Gran JT: The epidemiology of chronic generalized musculoskeletal pain. Best Pract Res Clin Rheumatol 2003; 17: 547–61
13. Moffett JK RG, Waddell G et al: Discussion Paper 129. Back pain: its management and costs to society, Centre for Health Economics, University of York , York, 1995
14. Picavet HSJ SJ, Smit HA: Prevelences and consequences of low back pain in the MORGEN-project 1993–1995. Bilthoven, NL, Rijksinstituut voor volksgezondheid en milieu, 1996
15. Andersson GB: Epidemiological features of chronic low-back pain. Lancet 1999; 354: 581–5
16. Hestbaek L, Leboeuf-Yde C, Manniche C: Low back pain: what is the long-term course? A review of studies of general patient populations. Eur Spine J 2003; 12: 149–65
17. Koes BW, van Tulder MW, Thomas S: Diagnosis and treatment of low back pain. Bmj 2006; 332: 1430–4
18. Frymoyer JW, Cats-Baril WL: An overview of the incidences and costs of low back pain. Orthop Clin North Am 1991; 22: 263–71

19. van Tulder M, Koes B, Bombardier C: Low back pain. Best Pract Res Clin Rheumatol 2002; 16: 761–75

20. Cedraschi C, Allaz AF: How to identify patients with a poor prognosis in daily clinical practice. Best Pract Res Clin Rheumatol 2005; 19: 577–91

21. Peters ML, Vlaeyen JW, Weber WE: The joint contribution of physical pathology, pain-related fear and catastrophizing to chronic back pain disability. Pain 2005; 113: 45–50

22. Manek NJ, MacGregor AJ: Epidemiology of back disorders: prevalence, risk factors, and prognosis. Curr Opin Rheumatol 2005; 17: 134–40

23. Diamond S, Borenstein D: Chronic low back pain in a working-age adult. Best Pract Res Clin Rheumatol 2006; 20: 707–20

24. Coderre TJ, Katz J, Vaccarino AL, Melzack R: Contribution of central neuroplasticity to pathological pain: review of clinical and experimental evidence. Pain 1993; 52: 259–85

25. Woolf CJ, Salter MW: Neuronal plasticity: increasing the gain in pain. Science 2000; 288: 1765–9

26. Melzack R, Coderre TJ, Katz J, Vaccarino AL: Central neuroplasticity and pathological pain. Ann N Y Acad Sci 2001; 933: 157–74

27. Wilder-Smith OH, Arendt-Nielsen L: Postoperative hyperalgesia: its clinical importance and relevance. Anesthesiology 2006; 104: 601–7

28. Bouhassira D, Chitour D, Villaneuva L, Le Bars D: The spinal transmission of nociceptive information: modulation by the caudal medulla. Neuroscience 1995; 69: 931–8

29. Price DD: Psychological and neural mechanisms of the affective dimension of pain. Science 2000; 288: 1769–72

30. Porreca F, Ossipov MH, Gebhart GF: Chronic pain and medullary descending facilitation. Trends Neurosci 2002; 25: 319–25

31. Gebhart GF: Descending modulation of pain. Neurosci Biobehav Rev 2004; 27: 729–37

32. Kosek E, Ordeberg G: Lack of pressure pain modulation by heterotopic noxious conditioning stimulation in patients with painful osteoarthritis before, but not following, surgical pain relief. Pain 2000; 88: 69–78

33. Edwards RR, Ness TJ, Weigent DA, Fillingim RB: Individual differences in diffuse noxious inhibitory controls (DNIC): association with clinical variables. Pain 2003; 106: 427–37

34. Edwards RR, Fillingim RB, Ness TJ: Age-related differences in endogenous pain modulation: a comparison of diffuse noxious inhibitory controls in healthy older and younger adults. Pain 2003; 101: 155–65

35. Edwards RR: Individual differences in endogenous pain modulation as a risk factor for chronic pain. Neurology 2005; 65: 437–43

36. Woolf CJ, Wall PD: Morphine-sensitive and morphine-insensitive actions of C-fibre input on the rat spinal cord. Neurosci Lett 1986; 64: 221–5

37. Tverskoy M, Oz Y, Isakson A, Finger J, Bradley EL, Jr., Kissin I: Preemptive effect of fentanyl and ketamine on postoperative pain and wound hyperalgesia. Anesth Analg 1994; 78: 205–9

38. Stubhaug A, Breivik H, Eide PK, Kreunen M, Foss A: Mapping of punctuate hyperalgesia around a surgical incision demonstrates that ketamine is a powerful suppressor of central sensitization to pain following surgery. Acta Anaesthesiol Scand 1997; 41: 1124–32

39. Moiniche S, Dahl JB, Erichsen CJ, Jensen LM, Kehlet H: Time course of subjective pain ratings, and wound and leg tenderness after hysterectomy. Acta Anaesthesiol Scand 1997; 41: 785–9

40. Lavand'homme P, De Kock M, Waterloos H: Intraoperative epidural analgesia combined with ketamine provides effective preventive analgesia in patients undergoing major digestive surgery. Anesthesiology 2005; 103: 813–20

41. De Kock M, Lavand'homme P, Waterloos H: 'Balanced analgesia' in the perioperative period: is there a place for ketamine? Pain 2001; 92: 373–80

42. De Kock M, Lavand'homme P, Waterloos H: The short-lasting analgesia and long-term antihyperalgesic effect of intrathecal clonidine in patients undergoing colonic surgery. Anesth Analg 2005; 101: 566–72, table of contents

43. Diatchenko L, Nackley AG, Slade GD, Fillingim RB, Maixner W: Idiopathic pain disorders–pathways of vulnerability. Pain 2006; 123: 226–30

44. Arendt-Nielsen L, Graven-Nielsen T: Central sensitization in fibromyalgia and other musculoskeletal disorders. Curr Pain Headache Rep 2003; 7: 355–61

45. O'Neill S, Manniche C, Graven-Nielsen T, Arendt-Nielsen L: Generalized deep-tissue hyperalgesia in patients with chronic low-back pain. Eur J Pain 2007; 11: 415–20

46. Lautenbacher S, Rollman GB: Possible deficiencies of pain modulation in fibromyalgia. Clin J Pain 1997; 13: 189–96

47. Gracely RH, Geisser ME, Giesecke T, Grant MA, Petzke F, Williams DA, Clauw DJ: Pain catastrophizing and neural responses to pain among persons with fibromyalgia. Brain 2004; 127: 835–43

48. Julien N, Goffaux P, Arsenault P, Marchand S: Widespread pain in fibromyalgia is related to a deficit of endogenous pain inhibition. Pain 2005; 114: 295–302

49. Maihofner C, Handwerker HO, Neundorfer B, Birklein F: Patterns of cortical reorganization in complex regional pain syndrome. Neurology 2003; 61: 1707–15

50. Verne GN, Price DD: Irritable bowel syndrome as a common precipitant of central sensitization. Curr Rheumatol Rep 2002; 4: 322–8

51. Shy ME, Frohman EM, So YT, Arezzo JC, Cornblath DR, Giuliani MJ, Kincaid JC, Ochoa JL, Parry GJ, Weimer LH: Quantitative sensory testing: report of the Therapeutics and Technology Assessment Subcommittee of the American Academy of Neurology. Neurology 2003; 60: 898–904

52. Chong PS, Cros DP: Technology literature review: quantitative sensory testing. Muscle Nerve 2004; 29: 734–47

53. Cruccu G, Anand P, Attal N, Garcia-Larrea L, Haanpaa M, Jorum E, Serra J, Jensen TS: EFNS guidelines on neuropathic pain assessment. Eur J Neurol 2004; 11: 153–62

54. Cruccu G, Truini A: Assessment of neuropathic pain. Neurol Sci 2006; 27 Suppl 4: s288–90

55. Zaslansky R, Yarnitsky D: Clinical applications of quantitative sensory testing (QST). J Neurol Sci 1998; 153: 215–38

56. Gruener G, Dyck PJ: Quantitative sensory testing: methodology, applications, and future directions. J Clin Neurophysiol 1994; 11: 568–83

57. Le Bars D, Dickenson AH, Besson JM: Diffuse noxious inhibitory controls (DNIC). II. Lack of effect on non-convergent neurones, supraspinal involvement and theoretical implications. Pain 1979; 6: 305–27

58. Le Bars D, Dickenson AH, Besson JM: Diffuse noxious inhibitory controls (DNIC). I. Effects on dorsal horn convergent neurones in the rat. Pain 1979; 6: 283–304

59. Granot M, Weissman-Fogel I, Crispel Y, Pud D, Granovsky Y, Sprecher E, Yarnitsky D: Determinants of endogenous analgesia magnitude in a diffuse noxious inhibitory control (DNIC) paradigm: do conditioning stimulus painfulness, gender and personality variables matter? Pain 2008; 136: 142–9

60. Pud D, Granovsky Y, Yarnitsky D: The methodology of experimentally induced diffuse noxious inhibitory control (DNIC)-like effect in humans. Pain 2009; 144: 16–9

61. Villanueva L: Diffuse Noxious Inhibitory Control (DNIC) as a tool for exploring dysfunction of endogenous pain modulatory systems. Pain 2009; 143: 161–2

62. Yarnitsky D, Arendt-Nielsen L, Bouhassira D, Edwards RR, Fillingim RB, Granot M, Hansson P, Lautenbacher S, Marchand S, Wilder-Smith O: Recommendations on terminology and practice of psychophysical DNIC testing. Eur J Pain 2010

63. Chua NH, Vissers KC, Arendt-Nielsen L, Wilder-Smith OH: Do diagnostic blocks have beneficial effects on pain processing? Reg Anesth Pain Med; 36: 317–21

64. Nir RR, Granovsky Y, Yarnitsky D, Sprecher E, Granot M: A psychophysical study of endogenous analgesia: the role of the conditioning pain in the induction and magnitude of conditioned pain modulation. Eur J Pain; 15: 491–7

65. Treister R, Eisenberg E, Gershon E, Haddad M, Pud D: Factors affecting - and relationships between-different modes of endogenous pain modulation in healthy volunteers. Eur J Pain; 14: 608–14

66. Yarnitsky D: Conditioned pain modulation (the diffuse noxious inhibitory control-like effect): its relevance for acute and chronic pain states. Curr Opin Anaesthesiol 2010; 23: 611–5

67. Rolke R, Baron R, Maier C, Tolle TR, Treede RD, Beyer A, Binder A, Birbaumer N, Birklein F, Botefur IC, Braune S, Flor H, Huge V, Klug R, Landwehrmeyer GB, Magerl W, Maihofner C, Rolko C, Schaub C, Scherens A, Sprenger T, Valet M, Wasserka B: Quantitative sensory testing in the German Research Network on Neuropathic Pain (DFNS): standardized protocol and reference values. Pain 2006; 123: 231–43

68. Rolke R, Magerl W, Campbell KA, Schalber C, Caspari S, Birklein F, Treede RD: Quantitative sensory testing: a comprehensive protocol for clinical trials. Eur J Pain 2006; 10: 77–88

69. Craig AD: How do you feel? Interoception: the sense of the physiological condition of the body. Nat Rev Neurosci 2002; 3: 655–66

70. Le Bars D: The whole body receptive field of dorsal horn multireceptive neurones. Brain Res Brain Res Rev 2002; 40: 29–44

71. McQuay HJ: Pre-emptive analgesia: a systematic review of clinical studies. Ann Med 1995; 27: 249–56

72. Wilder-Smith OH: Pre-emptive analgesia and surgical pain. Prog Brain Res 2000; 129: 505–24

73. Pogatzki-Zahn EM, Zahn PK: From preemptive to preventive analgesia. Curr Opin Anaesthesiol 2006; 19: 551–5

74. Grape S, Tramer MR: Do we need preemptive analgesia for the treatment of postoperative pain? Best Pract Res Clin Anaesthesiol 2007; 21: 51–63

75. Arendt-Nielsen L, Curatolo M, Drewes A: Human experimental pain models in drug development: translational pain research. Curr Opin Investig Drugs 2007; 8: 41–53
76. Max MB: Is mechanism-based pain treatment attainable? Clinical trial issues. J Pain 2000; 1: 2–9
77. Jensen TS, Baron R: Translation of symptoms and signs into mechanisms in neuropathic pain. Pain 2003; 102: 1–8
78. Baliki MN, Chialvo DR, Geha PY, Levy RM, Harden RN, Parrish TB, Apkarian AV: Chronic pain and the emotional brain: specific brain activity associated with spontaneous fluctuations of intensity of chronic back pain. J Neurosci 2006; 26: 12165–73
79. Greenspan JD: Quantitative assessment of neuropathic pain. Curr Pain Headache Rep 2001; 5: 107–13
80. Desmeules JA, Cedraschi C, Rapiti E, Baumgartner E, Finckh A, Cohen P, Dayer P, Vischer TL: Neurophysiologic evidence for a central sensitization in patients with fibromyalgia. Arthritis Rheum 2003; 48: 1420–9
81. Lowenstein L, Vardi Y, Deutsch M, Friedman M, Gruenwald I, Granot M, Sprecher E, Yarnitsky D: Vulvar vestibulitis severity–assessment by sensory and pain testing modalities. Pain 2004; 107: 47–53
82. Ordeberg G: Characterization of joint pain in human OA. Novartis Found Symp 2004; 260: 105–15; discussion 115–21, 277–9
83. Lang PM, Schober GM, Rolke R, Wagner S, Hilge R, Offenbacher M, Treede RD, Hoffmann U, Irnich D: Sensory neuropathy and signs of central sensitization in patients with peripheral arterial disease. Pain 2006; 124: 190–200
84. Ladda J, Straube A, Forderreuther S, Krause P, Eggert T: Quantitative sensory testing in cluster headache: increased sensory thresholds. Cephalalgia 2006; 26: 1043–50
85. Juhl GI, Jensen TS, Norholt SE, Svensson P: Central sensitization phenomena after third molar surgery: A quantitative sensory testing study. Eur J Pain 2007
86. Drewes AM, Schipper KP, Dimcevski G, Petersen P, Andersen OK, Gregersen H, Arendt-Nielsen L: Multi-modal induction and assessment of allodynia and hyperalgesia in the human oesophagus. Eur J Pain 2003; 7: 539–49
87. Drewes AM, Schipper KP, Dimcevski G, Petersen P, Andersen OK, Gregersen H, Arendt-Nielsen L: Multimodal assessment of pain in the esophagus: a new experimental model. Am J Physiol Gastrointest Liver Physiol 2002; 283: G95–103
88. Treede RD, Meyer RA, Raja SN, Campbell JN: Peripheral and central mechanisms of cutaneous hyperalgesia. Prog Neurobiol 1992; 38: 397–421
89. Treede RD, Rolke R, Andrews K, Magerl W: Pain elicited by blunt pressure: neurobiological basis and clinical relevance. Pain 2002; 98: 235–40
90. Walk D, Sehgal N, Moeller-Bertram T, Edwards RR, Wasan A, Wallace M, Irving G, Argoff C, Backonja MM: Quantitative sensory testing and mapping: a review of nonautomated quantitative methods for examination of the patient with neuropathic pain. Clin J Pain 2009; 25: 632–40
91. Arendt-Nielsen L, Yarnitsky D: Experimental and clinical applications of quantitative sensory testing applied to skin, muscles and viscera. J Pain 2009; 10: 556–72
92. Arendt-Nielsen L, Petersen-Felix S: Wind-up and neuroplasticity: is there a correlation to clinical pain? Eur J Anaesthesiol Suppl 1995; 10: 1–7
93. Pud D, Sprecher E, Yarnitsky D: Homotopic and heterotopic effects of endogenous analgesia in healthy volunteers. Neurosci Lett 2005; 380: 209–13

94. Arendt-Nielsen L, Sluka KA, Nie HL: Experimental muscle pain impairs descending inhibition. Pain 2008; 140: 465–71

95. Yarnitsky D, Crispel Y, Eisenberg E, Granovsky Y, Ben-Nun A, Sprecher E, Best LA, Granot M: Prediction of chronic post-operative pain: pre-operative DNIC testing identifies patients at risk. Pain 2008; 138: 22–8

96. Staud R, Robinson ME, Vierck CJ, Jr., Price DD: Diffuse noxious inhibitory controls (DNIC) attenuate temporal summation of second pain in normal males but not in normal females or fibromyalgia patients. Pain 2003; 101: 167–74

97. van den Broeke EN, van Rijn CM, Biurrun Manresa JA, Andersen OK, Arendt-Nielsen L, Wilder-Smith OH: Neurophysiological Correlates of Nociceptive Heterosynaptic Long-Term Potentiation in Humans. J Neurophysiol 2010

98. Adolph O, Koster S, Georgieff M, Bader S, Fohr KJ, Kammer T, Herrnberger B, Gron G: Xenon-induced changes in CNS sensitization to pain. Neuroimage 2010; 49: 720–30

99. Klein T, Stahn S, Magerl W, Treede RD: The role of heterosynaptic facilitation in long-term potentiation (LTP) of human pain sensation. Pain 2008; 139: 507–19

100. Klein T, Magerl W, Treede RD: Perceptual correlate of nociceptive long-term potentiation (LTP) in humans shares the time course of early-LTP. J Neurophysiol 2006; 96: 3551–5

101. Klein T, Magerl W, Hopf HC, Sandkuhler J, Treede RD: Perceptual correlates of nociceptive long-term potentiation and long-term depression in humans. J Neurosci 2004; 24: 964–71

102. Wilder-Smith OH: Changes in sensory processing after surgical nociception. Curr Rev Pain 2000; 4: 234–41

103. Edwards RR, Haythornthwaite JA, Tella P, Max MB, Raja S: Basal heat pain thresholds predict opioid analgesia in patients with postherpetic neuralgia. Anesthesiology 2006; 104: 1243–8

104. Geber C, Klein T, Azad S, Birklein F, Gierthmuhlen J, Huge V, Lauchart M, Nitzsche D, Stengel M, Valet M, Baron R, Maier C, Tolle T, Treede RD: Test-retest and interobserver reliability of quantitative sensory testing according to the protocol of the German Research Network on Neuropathic Pain (DFNS): a multi-centre study. Pain 2011; 152: 548–56

105. Kosek E, Ekholm J, Hansson P: Increased pressure pain sensibility in fibromyalgia patients is located deep to the skin but not restricted to muscle tissue. Pain 1995; 63: 335–9

106. Kosek E, Ekholm J, Hansson P: Pressure pain thresholds in different tissues in one body region. The influence of skin sensitivity in pressure algometry. Scand J Rehabil Med 1999; 31: 89–93

107. Rollman GB, Lautenbacher S: Sex differences in musculoskeletal pain. Clin J Pain 2001; 17: 20–4

108. Lautenbacher S, Rollman GB: Sex differences in responsiveness to painful and non-painful stimuli are dependent upon the stimulation method. Pain 1993; 53: 255–64

109. Lautenbacher S, Rollman GB, McCain GA: Multi-method assessment of experimental and clinical pain in patients with fibromyalgia. Pain 1994; 59: 45–53

110. Bisgaard T, Klarskov B, Rosenberg J, Kehlet H: Characteristics and prediction of early pain after laparoscopic cholecystectomy. Pain 2001; 90: 261–9

111. Chu LF, Clark DJ, Angst MS: Opioid tolerance and hyperalgesia in chronic pain patients after one month of oral morphine therapy: a preliminary prospective study. J Pain 2006; 7: 43–8

112. Mitchell LA, MacDonald RA, Brodie EE: Temperature and the cold pressor test. J Pain 2004; 5: 233–7

113. von Baeyer CL, Piira T, Chambers CT, Trapanotto M, Zeltzer LK: Guidelines for the cold pressor task as an experimental pain stimulus for use with children. J Pain 2005; 6: 218–27

114. Crombie IK, Davies HT, Macrae WA: Cut and thrust: antecedent surgery and trauma among patients attending a chronic pain clinic. Pain 1998; 76: 167–71

115. Bay-Nielsen M, Nilsson E, Nordin P, Kehlet H: Chronic pain after open mesh and sutured repair of indirect inguinal hernia in young males. Br J Surg 2004; 91: 1372–6

116. Bay-Nielsen M, Perkins FM, Kehlet H: Pain and functional impairment 1 year after inguinal herniorrhaphy: a nationwide questionnaire study. Ann Surg 2001; 233: 1–7

117. Callesen T, Bech K, Kehlet H: Prospective study of chronic pain after groin hernia repair. Br J Surg 1999; 86: 1528–31

118. Nikolajsen L, Kristensen AD, Thillemann TM, Jurik AG, Rasmussen T, Kehlet H, Jensen TS: Pain and somatosensory findings in patients 3 years after total hip arthroplasty. Eur J Pain 2009; 13: 576–81

119. Nikolajsen L, Brandsborg B, Lucht U, Jensen TS, Kehlet H: Chronic pain following total hip arthroplasty: a nationwide questionnaire study. Acta Anaesthesiol Scand 2006; 50: 495–500

120. Pluijms WA, Steegers MA, Verhagen AF, Scheffer GJ, Wilder-Smith OH: Chronic post-thoracotomy pain: a retrospective study. Acta Anaesthesiol Scand 2006; 50: 804–8

121. Edwards RR, Haythornthwaite JA, Smith MT, Klick B, Katz JN: Catastrophizing and depressive symptoms as prospective predictors of outcomes following total knee replacement. Pain Res Manag 2009; 14: 307–11

122. LaCroix-Fralish ML, Austin JS, Zheng FY, Levitin DJ, Mogil JS: Patterns of pain: meta-analysis of microarray studies of pain. Pain 2011; 152: 1888–98

123. LaCroix-Fralish ML, Mo G, Smith SB, Sotocinal SG, Ritchie J, Austin JS, Melmed K, Schorscher-Petcu A, Laferriere AC, Lee TH, Romanovsky D, Liao G, Behlke MA, Clark DJ, Peltz G, Seguela P, Dobretsov M, Mogil JS: The beta3 subunit of the Na+,K+-ATPase mediates variable nociceptive sensitivity in the formalin test. Pain 2009; 144: 294–302

124. Zhang J, Shi XQ, Echeverry S, Mogil JS, De Koninck Y, Rivest S: Expression of CCR2 in both resident and bone marrow-derived microglia plays a critical role in neuropathic pain. J Neurosci 2007; 27: 12396–406

125. Katz J, Seltzer Z: Transition from acute to chronic postsurgical pain: risk factors and protective factors. Expert Rev Neurother 2009; 9: 723–44

126. Campbell CM, Edwards RR, Carmona C, Uhart M, Wand G, Carteret A, Kim YK, Frost J, Campbell JN: Polymorphisms in the GTP cyclohydrolase gene (GCH1) are associated with ratings of capsaicin pain. Pain 2009; 141: 114–8

127. Mogil JS, Ritchie J, Sotocinal SG, Smith SB, Croteau S, Levitin DJ, Naumova AK: Screening for pain phenotypes: Analysis of three congenic mouse strains on a battery of nine nociceptive assays. Pain 2006

128. Stamer UM, Bayerer B, Stuber F: Genetics and variability in opioid response. Eur J Pain 2005; 9: 101–4

129. Katz J, Poleshuck EL, Andrus CH, Hogan LA, Jung BF, Kulick DI, Dworkin RH: Risk factors for acute pain and its persistence following breast cancer surgery. Pain 2005; 119: 16–25

130. Wilson SG, Bryant CD, Lariviere WR, Olsen MS, Giles BE, Chesler EJ, Mogil JS: The heritability of antinociception II: pharmacogenetic mediation of three over-the-counter analgesics in mice. J Pharmacol Exp Ther 2003; 305: 755–64

131. Wilson SG, Smith SB, Chesler EJ, Melton KA, Haas JJ, Mitton B, Strasburg K, Hubert L, Rodriguez-Zas SL, Mogil JS: The heritability of antinociception: common pharmacogenetic mediation of five neurochemically distinct analgesics. J Pharmacol Exp Ther 2003; 304: 547–59

132. Gursoy S, Erdal E, Herken H, Madenci E, Alasehirli B, Erdal N: Significance of catechol-O-methyltransferase gene polymorphism in fibromyalgia syndrome. Rheumatol Int 2003; 23: 104–7

133. Chesler EJ, Wilson SG, Lariviere WR, Rodriguez-Zas SL, Mogil JS: Identification and ranking of genetic and laboratory environment factors influencing a behavioral trait, thermal nociception, via computational analysis of a large data archive. Neurosci Biobehav Rev 2002; 26: 907–23

134. Wilson SG, Chesler EJ, Hain H, Rankin AJ, Schwarz JZ, Call SB, Murray MR, West EE, Teuscher C, Rodriguez-Zas S, Belknap JK, Mogil JS: Identification of quantitative trait loci for chemical/inflammatory nociception in mice. Pain 2002; 96: 385–91

135. Quartana PJ, Campbell CM, Edwards RR: Pain catastrophizing: a critical review. Expert Rev Neurother 2009; 9: 745–58

136. Papaioannou M, Skapinakis P, Damigos D, Mavreas V, Broumas G, Palgimesi A: The role of catastrophizing in the prediction of postoperative pain. Pain Med 2009; 10: 1452–9

137. Strulov L, Zimmer EZ, Granot M, Tamir A, Jakobi P, Lowenstein L: Pain catastrophizing, response to experimental heat stimuli, and post-cesarean section pain. J Pain 2007; 8: 273–9

138. Pavlin DJ, Sullivan MJ, Freund PR, Roesen K: Catastrophizing: a risk factor for postsurgical pain. Clin J Pain 2005; 21: 83–90

139. Latremoliere A, Woolf CJ: Central sensitization: a generator of pain hypersensitivity by central neural plasticity. J Pain 2009; 10: 895–926

140. Costigan M, Scholz J, Woolf CJ: Neuropathic pain: a maladaptive response of the nervous system to damage. Annu Rev Neurosci 2009; 32: 1–32

141. Vanegas H, Schaible HG: Descending control of persistent pain: inhibitory or facilitatory? Brain Res Brain Res Rev 2004; 46: 295–309

142. Vera-Portocarrero LP, Zhang ET, Ossipov MH, Xie JY, King T, Lai J, Porreca F: Descending facilitation from the rostral ventromedial medulla maintains nerve injury-induced central sensitization. Neuroscience 2006; 140: 1311–20

143. Sandkuhler J: Models and mechanisms of hyperalgesia and allodynia. Physiol Rev 2009; 89: 707–58

144. Sandkuhler J, Gruber-Schoffnegger D: Hyperalgesia by synaptic long-term potentiation (LTP): an update. Curr Opin Pharmacol 2011

145. Ruscheweyh R, Wilder-Smith O, Drdla R, Liu XG, Sandkuhler J: Long-term potentiation in spinal nociceptive pathways as a novel target for pain therapy. Mol Pain 2011; 7: 20

146. Sandkuhler J: Central sensitization versus synaptic long-term potentiation (LTP): a critical comment. J Pain 2010; 11: 798–800

147. Melzack R, Wall PD: Pain mechanisms: a new theory. Science 1965; 150: 971–9
148. Heinricher MM, Tavares I, Leith JL, Lumb BM: Descending control of nociception: Specificity, recruitment and plasticity. Brain Res Rev 2009; 60: 214–25
149. Apkarian AV, Baliki MN, Geha PY: Towards a theory of chronic pain. Prog Neurobiol 2009; 87: 81–97
150. Vera-Portocarrero LP, Xie JY, Kowal J, Ossipov MH, King T, Porreca F: Descending facilitation from the rostral ventromedial medulla maintains visceral pain in rats with experimental pancreatitis. Gastroenterology 2006; 130: 2155–64
151. Villanueva L, Le Bars D: The activation of bulbo-spinal controls by peripheral nociceptive inputs: diffuse noxious inhibitory controls. Biol Res 1995; 28: 113–25
152. Bouhassira D, Bing Z, Le Bars D: Studies of brain structures involved in diffuse noxious inhibitory controls in the rat: the rostral ventromedial medulla. J Physiol 1993; 463: 667–87
153. Morton CR, Maisch B, Zimmermann M: Diffuse noxious inhibitory controls of lumbar spinal neurons involve a supraspinal loop in the cat. Brain Res 1987; 410: 347–52
154. Finniss DG, Kaptchuk TJ, Miller F, Benedetti F: Biological, clinical, and ethical advances of placebo effects. Lancet 2010; 375: 686–95
155. Benedetti F: No prefrontal control, no placebo response. Pain 2010; 148: 357–8
156. Pollo A, Benedetti F: The placebo response: neurobiological and clinical issues of neurological relevance. Prog Brain Res 2009; 175: 283–94
157. Enck P, Benedetti F, Schedlowski M: New insights into the placebo and nocebo responses. Neuron 2008; 59: 195–206
158. Colloca L, Sigaudo M, Benedetti F: The role of learning in nocebo and placebo effects. Pain 2008; 136: 211–8
159. Apkarian AV, Bushnell MC, Treede RD, Zubieta JK: Human brain mechanisms of pain perception and regulation in health and disease. Eur J Pain 2005; 9: 463–84
160. Jensen KB, Kosek E, Petzke F, Carville S, Fransson P, Marcus H, Williams SC, Choy E, Giesecke T, Mainguy Y, Gracely R, Ingvar M: Evidence of dysfunctional pain inhibition in Fibromyalgia reflected in rACC during provoked pain. Pain 2009; 144: 95–100
161. Cervero F: Visceral pain-central sensitisation. Gut 2000; 47 Suppl 4: iv56–7; discussion iv58
162. Cervero F: Visceral hyperalgesia revisited. Lancet 2000; 356: 1127–8
163. Apkarian AV, Sosa Y, Sonty S, Levy RM, Harden RN, Parrish TB, Gitelman DR: Chronic back pain is associated with decreased prefrontal and thalamic gray matter density. J Neurosci 2004; 24: 10410–5
164. Truini A, Cruccu G: Pathophysiological mechanisms of neuropathic pain. Neurol Sci 2006; 27 Suppl 2: S179–82
165. Liu SS, Gerancher JC, Bainton BG, Kopacz DJ, Carpenter RL: The effects of electrical stimulation at different frequencies on perception and pain in human volunteers: epidural versus intravenous administration of fentanyl. Anesth Analg 1996; 82: 98–102
166. van der Burght M, Rasmussen SE, Arendt-Nielsen L, Bjerring P: Morphine does not affect laser induced warmth and pin prick pain thresholds. Acta Anaesthesiol Scand 1994; 38: 161–4
167. Gray BG, Dostrovsky JO: Descending inhibitory influences from periaqueductal gray, nucleus raphe magnus, and adjacent reticular formation. I. Effects on lumbar spinal cord nociceptive and nonnociceptive neurons. J Neurophysiol 1983; 49: 932–47

168. Kosek E, Hansson P: Modulatory influence on somatosensory perception from vibration and heterotopic noxious conditioning stimulation (HNCS) in fibromyalgia patients and healthy subjects. Pain 1997; 70: 41–51

169. Peters ML, Schmidt AJ, Van den Hout MA, Koopmans R, Sluijter ME: Chronic back pain, acute postoperative pain and the activation of diffuse noxious inhibitory controls (DNIC). Pain 1992; 50: 177–87

170. Granot M, Lowenstein L, Yarnitsky D, Tamir A, Zimmer EZ: Postcesarean section pain prediction by preoperative experimental pain assessment. Anesthesiology 2003; 98: 1422–6

171. Werner MU, Duun P, Kehlet H: Prediction of postoperative pain by preoperative nociceptive responses to heat stimulation. Anesthesiology 2004; 100: 115–9; discussion 5A

172. Dahl JB, Moiniche S: Pre-emptive analgesia. Br Med Bull 2004; 71: 13–27

173. Fletcher D: [Prevention of postoperative pain]. Ann Fr Anesth Reanim 1998; 17: 622–32

174. Katz J: Pre-emptive analgesia: evidence, current status and future directions. Eur J Anaesthesiol Suppl 1995; 10: 8–13

175. Wall PD: The prevention of postoperative pain. Pain 1988; 33: 289–90

176. Farasyn A, Meeusen R: The influence of non-specific low back pain on pressure pain thresholds and disability. Eur J Pain 2005; 9: 375–81

177. Strutton PH, Theodorou S, Catley M, McGregor AH, Davey NJ: Corticospinal excitability in patients with chronic low back pain. J Spinal Disord Tech 2005; 18: 420–4

178. Wilder-Smith OH: Chronic pain and surgery: a review of new insights from sensory testing. J Pain Palliat Care Pharmacother 2011; 25: 146–59

179. den Boer JJ, Oostendorp RA, Beems T, Munneke M, Evers AW: Continued disability and pain after lumbar disc surgery: the role of cognitive-behavioral factors. Pain 2006; 123: 45–52

180. den Boer JJ, Oostendorp RA, Beems T, Munneke M, Oerlemans M, Evers AW: A systematic review of bio-psychosocial risk factors for an unfavourable outcome after lumbar disc surgery. Eur Spine J 2006; 15: 527–36

181. Pielsticker A, Haag G, Zaudig M, Lautenbacher S: Impairment of pain inhibition in chronic tension-type headache. Pain 2005; 118: 215–23

182. Edwards RR, Ness TJ, Fillingim RB: Endogenous opioids, blood pressure, and diffuse noxious inhibitory controls: a preliminary study. Percept Mot Skills 2004; 99: 679–87

183. Diatchenko L, Slade GD, Nackley AG, Bhalang K, Sigurdsson A, Belfer I, Goldman D, Xu K, Shabalina SA, Shagin D, Max MB, Makarov SS, Maixner W: Genetic basis for individual variations in pain perception and the development of a chronic pain condition. Hum Mol Genet 2005; 14: 135–43

184. Dahl JB: Neuronal plasticity and pre-emptive analgesia: implications for the management of postoperative pain. Dan Med Bull 1994; 41: 434–42

185. Richmond CE, Bromley LM, Woolf CJ: Preoperative morphine pre-empts postoperative pain. Lancet 1993; 342: 73–5

186. Richebe P, Rivat C, Laulin JP, Maurette P, Simonnet G: Ketamine improves the management of exaggerated postoperative pain observed in perioperative fentanyl-treated rats. Anesthesiology 2005; 102: 421–8

187. Visser E, Schug SA: The role of ketamine in pain management. Biomed Pharmacother 2006; 60: 341–8

188. Annetta MG, Iemma D, Garisto C, Tafani C, Proietti R: Ketamine: new indications for an old drug. Curr Drug Targets 2005; 6: 789–94

189. Bell RF, Dahl JB, Moore RA, Kalso E: Peri-operative ketamine for acute post-operative pain: a quantitative and qualitative systematic review (Cochrane review). Acta Anaesthesiol Scand 2005; 49: 1405–28

190. Elia N, Tramer MR: Ketamine and postoperative pain–a quantitative systematic review of randomised trials. Pain 2005; 113: 61–70

191. Himmelseher S, Durieux ME: Ketamine for perioperative pain management. Anesthesiology 2005; 102: 211–20

192. Bell RF, Dahl JB, Moore RA, Kalso E: Perioperative ketamine for acute postoperative pain. Cochrane Database Syst Rev 2006: CD004603

193. Celestin J, Edwards RR, Jamison RN: Pretreatment psychosocial variables as predictors of outcomes following lumbar surgery and spinal cord stimulation: a systematic review and literature synthesis. Pain Med 2009; 10: 639–53

194. Freynhagen R, Rolke R, Baron R, Tolle TR, Rutjes AK, Schu S, Treede RD: Pseudoradicular and radicular low-back pain - A disease continuum rather than different entities? Answers from quantitative sensory testing. Pain 2007; 135: 65–74

195. Freynhagen R, Baron R, Gockel U, Tolle TR: painDETECT: a new screening questionnaire to identify neuropathic components in patients with back pain. Curr Med Res Opin 2006; 22: 1911–20

196. Freynhagen R, Baron R, Tolle T, Stemmler E, Gockel U, Stevens M, Maier C: Screening of neuropathic pain components in patients with chronic back pain associated with nerve root compression: a prospective observational pilot study (MIPORT). Curr Med Res Opin 2006; 22: 529–37

197. Christoph T, Schiene K, Englberger W, Parsons CG, Chizh BA: The antiallodynic effect of NMDA antagonists in neuropathic pain outlasts the duration of the in vivo NMDA antagonism. Neuropharmacology 2006; 51: 12–7

198. Woolf CJ: Dissecting out mechanisms responsible for peripheral neuropathic pain: implications for diagnosis and therapy. Life Sci 2004; 74: 2605–10

199. Jorum E, Warncke T, Stubhaug A: Cold allodynia and hyperalgesia in neuropathic pain: the effect of N-methyl-D-aspartate (NMDA) receptor antagonist ketamine–a double-blind, cross-over comparison with alfentanil and placebo. Pain 2003; 101: 229–35

200. Gottrup H, Andersen J, Arendt-Nielsen L, Jensen TS: Psychophysical examination in patients with post-mastectomy pain. Pain 2000; 87: 275–84

201. Sayed-Noor AS, Englund E, Wretenberg P, Sjoden GO: Pressure-pain threshold algometric measurement in patients with greater trochanteric pain after total hip arthroplasty. Clin J Pain 2008; 24: 232–6

202. Bessiere B, Laboureyras E, Chateauraynaud J, Laulin JP, Simonnet G: A single nitrous oxide (N2O) exposure leads to persistent alleviation of neuropathic pain in rats. J Pain 2010; 11: 13–23

203. Richebe P, Rivat C, Creton C, Laulin JP, Maurette P, Lemaire M, Simonnet G: Nitrous oxide revisited: evidence for potent antihyperalgesic properties. Anesthesiology 2005; 103: 845–54

204. Echevarria G, Elgueta F, Fierro C, Bugedo D, Faba G, Iniguez-Cuadra R, Munoz HR, Cortinez LI: Nitrous oxide (N(2)O) reduces postoperative opioid-induced hyperalgesia after remifentanil-propofol anaesthesia in humans. Br J Anaesth 2011; 107: 959–65

205. Bessiere B, Richebe P, Laboureyras E, Laulin JP, Contarino A, Simonnet G: Nitrous oxide (N2O) prevents latent pain sensitization and long-term anxiety-like behavior in pain and opioid-experienced rats. Neuropharmacology 2007; 53: 733–40

206. Yarnitsky D, Granot M, Nahman-Averbuch H, Khamaisi M, Granovsky Y: Conditioned pain modulation predicts duloxetine efficacy in painful diabetic neuropathy. Pain 2012; 153: 1193–8

207. Verhaak PF, Kerssens JJ, Dekker J, Sorbi MJ, Bensing JM: Prevalence of chronic benign pain disorder among adults: a review of the literature. Pain 1998; 77: 231–9

208. Reid KJ, Harker J, Bala MM, Truyers C, Kellen E, Bekkering GE, Kleijnen J: Epidemiology of chronic non-cancer pain in Europe: narrative review of prevalence, pain treatments and pain impact. Curr Med Res Opin; 27: 449–62

209. Blyth FM, March LM, Brnabic AJ, Jorm LR, Williamson M, Cousins MJ: Chronic pain in Australia: a prevalence study. Pain 2001; 89: 127–34

210. Turk DC: Clinical effectiveness and cost-effectiveness of treatments for patients with chronic pain. Clin J Pain 2002; 18: 355–65

211. Collins SL, Moore RA, McQuayHj, Wiffen P: Antidepressants and anticonvulsants for diabetic neuropathy and postherpetic neuralgia: a quantitative systematic review. J Pain Symptom Manage 2000; 20: 449–58

212. Dvorak J, Gauchat MH, Valach L: The outcome of surgery for lumbar disc herniation. I. A 4–17 years' follow-up with emphasis on somatic aspects. Spine 1988; 13: 1418–22

213. Lehmann TR, Spratt KF, Tozzi JE, Weinstein JN, Reinarz SJ, el-Khoury GY, Colby H: Long-term follow-up of lower lumbar fusion patients. Spine 1987; 12: 97–104

214. North RB, Campbell JN, James CS, Conover-Walker MK, Wang H, Piantadosi S, Rybock JD, Long DM: Failed back surgery syndrome: 5-year follow-up in 102 patients undergoing repeated operation. Neurosurgery 1991; 28: 685–90; discussion 690–1

215. Woolf CJ, Max MB: Mechanism-based pain diagnosis: issues for analgesic drug development. Anesthesiology 2001; 95: 241–9

216. Woolf CJ, Bennett GJ, Doherty M, Dubner R, Kidd B, Koltzenburg M, Lipton R, Loeser JD, Payne R, Torebjork E: Towards a mechanism-based classification of pain? Pain 1998; 77: 227–9

217. Boivie J: Central pain and the role of quantitative sensory testing (QST) in research and diagnosis. Eur J Pain 2003; 7: 339–43

218. Bradley LA, McKendree-Smith NL: Central nervous system mechanisms of pain in fibromyalgia and other musculoskeletal disorders: behavioral and psychologic treatment approaches. Curr Opin Rheumatol 2002; 14: 45–51

219. Nijs J, Van Houdenhove B: From acute musculoskeletal pain to chronic widespread pain and fibromyalgia: application of pain neurophysiology in manual therapy practice. Man Ther 2009; 14: 3–12

220. Burgmer M, Gaubitz M, Konrad C, Wrenger M, Hilgart S, Heuft G, Pfleiderer B: Decreased gray matter volumes in the cingulo-frontal cortex and the amygdala in patients with fibromyalgia. Psychosom Med 2009; 71: 566–73

221. Burgmer M, Pogatzki-Zahn E, Gaubitz M, Wessoleck E, Heuft G, Pfleiderer B: Altered brain activity during pain processing in fibromyalgia. Neuroimage 2009; 44: 502–8

222. Burgmer M, Pogatzki-Zahn E, Gaubitz M, Stuber C, Wessoleck E, Heuft G, Pfleiderer B: Fibromyalgia unique temporal brain activation during experimental pain: a controlled fMRI Study. J Neural Transm 2010; 117: 123–31

223. Leffler AS, Kosek E, Lerndal T, Nordmark B, Hansson P: Somatosensory perception and function of diffuse noxious inhibitory controls (DNIC) in patients suffering from rheumatoid arthritis. Eur J Pain 2002; 6: 161–76

224. Edwards RR, Bingham CO, 3rd, Bathon J, Haythornthwaite JA: Catastrophizing and pain in arthritis, fibromyalgia, and other rheumatic diseases. Arthritis Rheum 2006; 55: 325–32

225. Bradley LA, Kersh BC, DeBerry JJ, Deutsch G, Alarcon GA, McLain DA: Lessons from fibromyalgia: abnormal pain sensitivity in knee osteoarthritis. Novartis Found Symp 2004; 260: 258–70; discussion 270–9

226. Rossel P, Pedersen P, Niddam D, Arendt-Nielsen L, Chen AC, Drewes AM: Cerebral response to electric stimulation of the colon and abdominal skin in healthy subjects and patients with irritable bowel syndrome. Scand J Gastroenterol 2001; 36: 1259–66

227. Wilder-Smith CH, Schindler D, Lovblad K, Redmond SM, Nirkko A: Brain functional magnetic resonance imaging of rectal pain and activation of endogenous inhibitory mechanisms in irritable bowel syndrome patient subgroups and healthy controls. Gut 2004; 53: 1595–601

228. Dimcevski G, Staahl C, Andersen SD, Thorsgaard N, Funch-Jensen P, Arendt-Nielsen L, Drewes AM: Assessment of experimental pain from skin, muscle, and esophagus in patients with chronic pancreatitis. Pancreas 2007; 35: 22–9

229. Dimcevski G, Sami SA, Funch-Jensen P, Le Pera D, Valeriani M, Arendt-Nielsen L, Drewes AM: Pain in chronic pancreatitis: the role of reorganization in the central nervous system. Gastroenterology 2007; 132: 1546–56

230. Giamberardino MA, Affaitati G, Lerza R, Lapenna D, Costantini R, Vecchiet L: Relationship between pain symptoms and referred sensory and trophic changes in patients with gallbladder pathology. Pain 2005; 114: 239–49

231. Chen AC, Dworkin SF, Haug J, Gehrig J: Human pain responsivity in a tonic pain model: psychological determinants. Pain 1989; 37: 143–60

232. Bouhassira D, Danziger N, Attal N, Guirimand F: Comparison of the pain suppressive effects of clinical and experimental painful conditioning stimuli. Brain 2003; 126: 1068–78

233. Modir JG, Wallace MS: Human experimental pain models 2: the cold pressor model. Methods Mol Biol 2010; 617: 165–8

234. Small DM, Apkarian AV: Increased taste intensity perception exhibited by patients with chronic back pain. Pain 2006; 120: 124–30

235. de Klaver MJ, van Rijn MA, Marinus J, Soede W, de Laat JA, van Hilten JJ: Hyperacusis in patients with complex regional pain syndrome related dystonia. J Neurol Neurosurg Psychiatry 2007; 78: 1310–3

236. Apkarian AV, Sosa Y, Krauss BR, Thomas PS, Fredrickson BE, Levy RE, Harden RN, Chialvo DR: Chronic pain patients are impaired on an emotional decision-making task. Pain 2004; 108: 129–36

237. Jongsma ML, Postma SA, Souren P, Arns M, Gordon E, Vissers K, Wilder-Smith O, van Rijn CM, van Goor H: Neurodegenerative properties of chronic pain: cognitive decline in patients with chronic pancreatitis. PLoS One 2011; 6: e23363

238. Tandon OP, Kumar S: P3 event related cerebral evoked potential in chronic pain patients. Indian J Physiol Pharmacol 1993; 37: 51–5

239. Maihofner C, Handwerker HO, Neundorfer B, Birklein F: Cortical reorganization during recovery from complex regional pain syndrome. Neurology 2004; 63: 693–701

240. Eisenberg E, Chistyakov AV, Yudashkin M, Kaplan B, Hafner H, Feinsod M: Evidence for cortical hyperexcitability of the affected limb representation area in CRPS: a psychophysical and transcranial magnetic stimulation study. Pain 2005; 113: 99–105

241. Drewes AM, Gratkowski M, Sami SA, Dimcevski G, Funch-Jensen P, Arendt-Nielsen L: Is the pain in chronic pancreatitis of neuropathic origin? Support from EEG studies during experimental pain. World J Gastroenterol 2008; 14: 4020–7

242. Frokjaer JB, Bouwense SA, Olesen SS, Lundager FH, Eskildsen SF, van Goor H, Wilder-Smith OH, Drewes AM: Reduced Cortical Thickness of Brain Areas Involved in Pain Processing in Patients with Chronic Pancreatitis. Clin Gastroenterol Hepatol 2011

243. Frokjaer JB, Olesen SS, Gram M, Yavarian Y, Bouwense SA, Wilder-Smith OH, Drewes AM: Altered brain microstructure assessed by diffusion tensor imaging in patients with chronic pancreatitis. Gut 2011; 60: 1554–62

244. Olesen SS, Brock C, Krarup AL, Funch-Jensen P, Arendt-Nielsen L, Wilder-Smith OH, Drewes AM: Descending inhibitory pain modulation is impaired in patients with chronic pancreatitis. Clin Gastroenterol Hepatol 2010; 8: 724–30

245. Olesen SS, Frokjaer JB, Lelic D, Valeriani M, Drewes AM: Pain-associated adaptive cortical reorganisation in chronic pancreatitis. Pancreatology 2010; 10: 742–51

246. Olesen SS, Hansen TM, Graversen C, Steimle K, Wilder-Smith OH, Drewes AM: Slowed EEG rhythmicity in patients with chronic pancreatitis: evidence of abnormal cerebral pain processing? Eur J Gastroenterol Hepatol 2011; 23: 418–24

247. Apkarian AV, Hashmi JA, Baliki MN: Pain and the brain: specificity and plasticity of the brain in clinical chronic pain. Pain 2011; 152: S49–64

248. Baliki MN, Baria AT, Apkarian AV: The cortical rhythms of chronic back pain. J Neurosci 2011; 31: 13981–90

249. Baliki MN, Schnitzer TJ, Bauer WR, Apkarian AV: Brain morphological signatures for chronic pain. PLoS One 2011; 6: e26010

250. Diers M, Koeppe C, Yilmaz P, Thieme K, Markela-Lerenc J, Schiltenwolf M, van Ackern K, Flor H: Pain ratings and somatosensory evoked responses to repetitive intramuscular and intracutaneous stimulation in fibromyalgia syndrome. J Clin Neurophysiol 2008; 25: 153–60

251. Lutz J, Jager L, de Quervain D, Krauseneck T, Padberg F, Wichnalek M, Beyer A, Stahl R, Zirngibl B, Morhard D, Reiser M, Schelling G: White and gray matter abnormalities in the brain of patients with fibromyalgia: a diffusion-tensor and volumetric imaging study. Arthritis Rheum 2008; 58: 3960–9

252. Schmidt-Wilcke T: Variations in brain volume and regional morphology associated with chronic pain. Curr Rheumatol Rep 2008; 10: 467–74

253. Nebel MB, Gracely RH: Neuroimaging of fibromyalgia. Rheum Dis Clin North Am 2009; 35: 313–27

254. Pujol J, Lopez-Sola M, Ortiz H, Vilanova JC, Harrison BJ, Yucel M, Soriano-Mas C, Cardoner N, Deus J: Mapping brain response to pain in fibromyalgia patients using temporal analysis of FMRI. PLoS One 2009; 4: e5224

255. Lotze M, Flor H, Grodd W, Larbig W, Birbaumer N: Phantom movements and pain. An fMRI study in upper limb amputees. Brain 2001; 124: 2268–77

256. Karl A, Muhlnickel W, Kurth R, Flor H: Neuroelectric source imaging of steady-state movement-related cortical potentials in human upper extremity amputees with and without phantom limb pain. Pain 2004; 110: 90–102

257. Karl A, Diers M, Flor H: P300-amplitudes in upper limb amputees with and without phantom limb pain in a visual oddball paradigm. Pain 2004; 110: 40–8

258. Flor H, Nikolajsen L, Staehelin Jensen T: Phantom limb pain: a case of maladaptive CNS plasticity? Nat Rev Neurosci 2006; 7: 873–81

259. Flor H: Maladaptive plasticity, memory for pain and phantom limb pain: review and suggestions for new therapies. Expert Rev Neurother 2008; 8: 809–18

260. Brinkert W, Dimcevski G, Arendt-Nielsen L, Drewes AM, Wilder-Smith OH: Dysmenorrhoea is associated with hypersensitivity in the sigmoid colon and rectum. Pain 2007

261. Maixner W, Fillingim R, Booker D, Sigurdsson A: Sensitivity of patients with painful temporomandibular disorders to experimentally evoked pain. Pain 1995; 63: 341–51

262. Wieseler-Frank J, Maier SF, Watkins LR: Glial activation and pathological pain. Neurochemistry International 2004; 45: 389–95

263. Wieseler-Frank J, Maier SF, Watkins LR: Immune-to-brain communication dynamically modulates pain: physiological and pathological consequences. Brain Behav Immun 2005; 19: 104–11

264. Angst MS, Clark JD: Opioid-induced hyperalgesia: a qualitative systematic review. Anesthesiology 2006; 104: 570–87

265. Chang G, Chen L, Mao J: Opioid tolerance and hyperalgesia. Med Clin North Am 2007; 91: 199–211

266. Koppert W: [Opioid-induced analgesia and hyperalgesia]. Schmerz 2005; 19: 386–90, 392–4

267. Mao J: Opioid-induced abnormal pain sensitivity. Curr Pain Headache Rep 2006; 10: 67–70

268. Mercadante S, Arcuri E: Hyperalgesia and opioid switching. Am J Hosp Palliat Care 2005; 22: 291–4

269. Simonnet G, Rivat C: Opioid-induced hyperalgesia: abnormal or normal pain? Neuroreport 2003; 14: 1–7

270. Banks WA, Watkins LR: Mediation of chronic pain: not by neurons alone. Pain 2006; 124: 1–2

271. Twining CM, Sloane EM, Schoeniger DK, Milligan ED, Martin D, Marsh H, Maier SF, Watkins LR: Activation of the spinal cord complement cascade might contribute to mechanical allodynia induced by three animal models of spinal sensitization. J Pain 2005; 6: 174–83

272. Watkins LR, Maier SF: Immune regulation of central nervous system functions: from sickness responses to pathological pain. J Intern Med 2005; 257: 139–55

273. Milligan ED, Watkins LR: Pathological and protective roles of glia in chronic pain. Nat Rev Neurosci 2009; 10: 23–36

274. Koppert W, Sittl R, Scheuber K, Alsheimer M, Schmelz M, Schuttler J: Differential modulation of remifentanil-induced analgesia and postinfusion hyperalgesia by S-ketamine and clonidine in humans. Anesthesiology 2003; 99: 152–9

275. Compton P, Athanasos P, Elashoff D: Withdrawal hyperalgesia after acute opioid physical dependence in nonaddicted humans: a preliminary study. J Pain 2003; 4: 511–9

276. Ram KC, Eisenberg E, Haddad M, Pud D: Oral opioid use alters DNIC but not cold pain perception in patients with chronic pain - new perspective of opioid-induced hyperalgesia. Pain 2008; 139: 431–8

277. Rommel O, Malin JP, Zenz M, Janig W: Quantitative sensory testing, neurophysiological and psychological examination in patients with complex regional pain syndrome and hemisensory deficits. Pain 2001; 93: 279–93

278. Bryan AS, Klenerman L, Bowsher D: The diagnosis of reflex sympathetic dystrophy using an algometer. J Bone Joint Surg Br 1991; 73: 644–6

279. Vatine JJ, Tsenter J, Nirel R: Experimental pressure pain in patients with complex regional pain syndrome, Type I (reflex sympathetic dystrophy). Am J Phys Med Rehabil 1998; 77: 382–7

280. Birklein F, Riedl B, Sieweke N, Weber M, Neundorfer B: Neurological findings in complex regional pain syndromes–analysis of 145 cases. Acta Neurol Scand 2000; 101: 262–9

281. Chesterton LS, Barlas P, Foster NE, Baxter GD, Wright CC: Gender differences in pressure pain threshold in healthy humans. Pain 2003; 101: 259–66

282. Arendt-Nielsen L, Bajaj P, Drewes AM: Visceral pain: gender differences in response to experimental and clinical pain. Eur J Pain 2004; 8: 465–72

283. Craft RM, Mogil JS, Aloisi AM: Sex differences in pain and analgesia: the role of gonadal hormones. Eur J Pain 2004; 8: 397–411

284. Fillingim RB, Gear RW: Sex differences in opioid analgesia: clinical and experimental findings. Eur J Pain 2004; 8: 413–25

285. Mayer EA, Berman S, Chang L, Naliboff BD: Sex-based differences in gastrointestinal pain. Eur J Pain 2004; 8: 451–63

286. France CR, Froese SA, Stewart JC: Altered central nervous system processing of noxious stimuli contributes to decreased nociceptive responding in individuals at risk for hypertension. Pain 2002; 98: 101–8

287. Park KM, Max MB, Robinovitz E, Gracely RH, Bennett GJ: Effects of intravenous ketamine, alfentanil, or placebo on pain, pinprick hyperalgesia, and allodynia produced by intradermal capsaicin in human subjects. Pain 1995; 63: 163–72

288. Richebe P, Rivat C, Rivalan B, Maurette P, Simonnet G: [Low doses ketamine: antihyperalgesic drug, non-analgesic]. Ann Fr Anesth Reanim 2005; 24: 1349–59

289. Klein T, Magerl W, Nickel U, Hopf HC, Sandkuhler J, Treede RD: Effects of the NMDA-receptor antagonist ketamine on perceptual correlates of long-term potentiation within the nociceptive system. Neuropharmacology 2007; 52: 655–61

290. Nikolajsen L, Hansen CL, Nielsen J, Keller J, Arendt-Nielsen L, Jensen TS: The effect of ketamine on phantom pain: a central neuropathic disorder maintained by peripheral input. Pain 1996; 67: 69–77

291. Ilkjaer S, Petersen KL, Brennum J, Wernberg M, Dahl JB: Effect of systemic N-methyl-D-aspartate receptor antagonist (ketamine) on primary and secondary hyperalgesia in humans. Br J Anaesth 1996; 76: 829–34

292. Felsby S, Nielsen J, Arendt-Nielsen L, Jensen TS: NMDA receptor blockade in chronic neuropathic pain: a comparison of ketamine and magnesium chloride. Pain 1996; 64: 283–91

293. Remerand F, Le Tendre C, Baud A, Couvret C, Pourrat X, Favard L, Laffon M, Fusciardi J: The early and delayed analgesic effects of ketamine after total hip arthroplasty: a prospective, randomized, controlled, double-blind study. Anesth Analg 2009; 109: 1963–71

294. Sen H, Sizlan A, Yanarates O, Emirkadi H, Ozkan S, Dagli G, Turan A: A comparison of gabapentin and ketamine in acute and chronic pain after hysterectomy. Anesth Analg 2009; 109: 1645–50

295. Joly V, Richebe P, Guignard B, Fletcher D, Maurette P, Sessler DI, Chauvin M: Remifentanil-induced postoperative hyperalgesia and its prevention with small-dose ketamine. Anesthesiology 2005; 103: 147–55

296. Olesen SS, Bouwense SA, Wilder-Smith OH, van Goor H, Drewes AM: Pregabalin reduces pain in patients with chronic pancreatitis in a randomized, controlled trial. Gastroenterology 2011; 141: 536–43

297. Buscher HC, Jansen JJ, van Goor H: Bilateral thoracoscopic splanchnicectomy in patients with chronic pancreatitis. Scand J Gastroenterol Suppl 1999; 230: 29–34

298. Buscher HC, Jansen JB, van Dongen R, Bleichrodt RP, van Goor H: Long-term results of bilateral thoracoscopic splanchnicectomy in patients with chronic pancreatitis. Br J Surg 2002; 89: 158–62

299. Bhatia M, Brady M, Shokuhi S, Christmas S, Neoptolemos JP, Slavin J: Inflammatory mediators in acute pancreatitis. J Pathol 2000; 190: 117–25

300. Flor H, Birbaumer N: Phantom limb pain: cortical plasticity and novel therapeutic approaches. Curr Opin Anaesthesiol 2000; 13: 561–4

About the Author

Dr. Wilder-Smith is Associate Professor for Pain and Nociception, and Consultant in Anaesthesiology and Pain Medicine at the Department of Anaesthesiology, Pain and Palliative Medicine at Radboud University Nijmegen Medical Centre, Nijmegen, Netherlands. He is associated with the Donders Centre for Cognition and Neuroscience at Radboud University Nijmegen, Netherlands as Head of the Pain and Nociception Neuroscience Research Group (PNNRG) and Principal Investigator. Furthermore he is Visiting Professor at the Centre for Sensory Motor interaction (SMI), Department of Health Science and Technology, Aalborg University, Denmark.

Dr. Wilder-Smith's main research areas cover chronic pain, particularly visceral and neuropathic, and chronic pain development, particularly after surgery. His overarching interest lies in elucidating patterns and mechanisms of altered CNS processing (cognitive, sensory, motor) in both experimental and clinical pain models. He actively participates in the establishment of translational pain models via parallel animal, human volunteer and patient models. In the areas of clinical research and patient care his interests include objective pain diagnostics such as quantitative sensory testing and electroencephalography, pain and treatment outcome prediction for individualised pain management, and the investigation of pharmacological and non-pharmacological treatment and prevention of chronic pain.

Dr. Wilder-Smith has published over 150 international peer-reviewed papers, written some 20 book chapters and held over 100 invited international lectures. He is a lecturer for the MSc courses for Interdisciplinary Pain Medicine at Vienna and Barcelona Universities, and is a member of the curriculum commission for the Pain MSc course at Vienna University. He has been opponent or supervisor for multiple PhDs, and is associate editor for the European Journal of Pain. Dr. Wilder-Smith is a regular reviewer for international pain and anaesthesia journals and has been expert reviewer for German (BMBF), Dutch (NWO). Swiss (SNF) and Austrian (ONBJF) scientific grant funding agencies.

Apart from his role as chief organiser of the 2013 IASP Research Symposium, Dr. Wilder-Smith is member of the Scientific Committee and Subcommittee for Research of the European Federation of IASP Chapters (EFIC); for 2013 he was Scientific Programme Committee Chairman for the biannual international EFIC Pain in Europe Congress in Florence.

www.ingramcontent.com/pod-product-compliance
Lightning Source LLC
Chambersburg PA
CBHW060445240326
41598CB00087B/3484